Somatic Intelligence
Volume 6

Opposing Gravity

How to Recognize and Recover from Head Injuries

(from a patient's perspective)

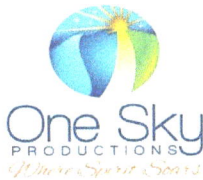

For information contact :

One Sky Productions

P.O. Box 150954

San Rafael, CA 94915

info@neurosomatics.info

www.neurosomatics.net

Book and Cover design by Suresha Hill

First Edition: January 2019

Table of Contents

Acknowledgments

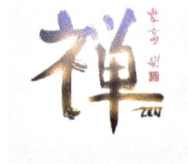

Many thanks to all the talented teachers and practitioners
who have made a world of difference in my body's ability to heal.
Without you I wouldn't be able to write this book or lead a joyful life.

Forward

Bruno Chikly, MD, DO (French)

It is always a pleasure to introduce a book written with so much enthusiasm and passion. Patients with traumatic brain injury or craniocerebral trauma (which are trauma involving the cranium and intracranial structures) are numerous and present often difficult problems that are usually not adequately helped by surgery nor medications. Cranial trauma and its sequelae can be one of the most challenging areas of the healthcare system today.

The causes of TBI are numerous. On the top of the list are motor vehicle accidents, firearm injuries, and falls. Motor vehicle accidents alone account for almost half of the TBIs in the United States. Overall the direct cost of care for adults with TBI in the United States excluding inpatient care has been estimated at more than $25 billion annually. A noninvasive and efficient approach to treat the central nervous system would be welcome for these typically very sensitive patients.

Brain Therapy was developed to fulfill the need for these patients. It is taught to medical doctors, osteopaths, chiropractors, physical therapists, occupational therapists, nurses, and numerous other manual therapy professions. The brain is the most profound of organs, yet is often overlooked in manual therapy. The central nervous system is an "intelligent" tissue and responds to subtle information such as our physical touch. Specific manual treatment of the central nervous system (CNS) often has far- reaching effects throughout the whole body, but advanced training is required to be able to properly assess and treat this system. A.T. Still, the father of osteopathy, said, "Of all the parts of the body of man to be well studied, the brain should be the most attractive." [1,2].

Brain Therapy is an advanced-level curriculum explores the brain and spinal cord structures. Students will learn specific techniques to release brain-centered restrictions as well as the damaging effects that these restrictions cause. These are advanced classes that use a slightly different paradigm by working extensively with brain structures. Manual therapists have to be made aware their hands have the potential to interact and discern these different structures. Dr. W. G. Sutherland, creator of osteopathy in the cranial field explained, "I know that the normal brain lives, thinks, and moves within its own specific membranous articular mechanism"

It takes a few classes to be able to address all these structures, but even the very first level of this curriculum may help therapists immediately improve their clinical results. These central nervous system structures are habitually unaddressed tissue lesions as well as key tissue restrictions. The body frequently aligns itself around these precise structures, and if injured, these CNS lesions often become unaddressed key or dominant tissue restrictions. This means if you can successfully treat these lesions, many other related problems in the body will also be treated and the patient will feel much better, much more functional and comfortable.

To efficiently work on the brain and spinal cord we need to address all the following structures:
1- Bones (intra- and inter-osseous lesions)
2- Membranes (dura, arachnoid, pia, basal membrane, etc.)
3- Three levels of cerebrospinal fluid: intraventricular, parenchymal and subarachnoid spaces with the cisternae.
4- Parenchyma grey matter: cortical, sub-cortical (nuclei) lesions
5- White matter lesions (commissures, association fibers and projections fibers)
6- Brain vasculature: veins, arteries and lymphatics
7- Peripheral nervous system: somatic and autonomic nerves
8- Cells, neurotransmitters and smaller lesions may also need to be addressed.
9- Other lesions (chemical, electromagnetic, emotional etc.)

The brain is extraordinary. 50% or more of the genetic code is allocated to the central nervous system. Each second of the first six months of gestation two million new connections are created in the brain. The rapidity at which neural connections are made during the first 18 months of life is astonishing. Undoubtedly, a tissue of this extraordinary nobility is worthy of our attention. I would like every student to appreciate and admire as I do the beauty and sensitivity of the central nervous system, and be amazed at the results with patients when the brain or spinal cord is touched with respect and wisdom.

Dr. Bruno Chikly,
Scottsdale, AZ; December 2018

References:

1. Still AT, Philosophy of Osteopathy, AT Still; Kirksville, MO Pub., 1899, p 47.

2. Still AT, The Philosophy and Mechanical Principles of Osteopathy, Kansas, MO Hudson-Kimberly Pub. Co, 1902, p 40.

3. Sutherland WG, "The Cranial Bowl", Free Press, First Edition 1939, reprint 1994, p. 51

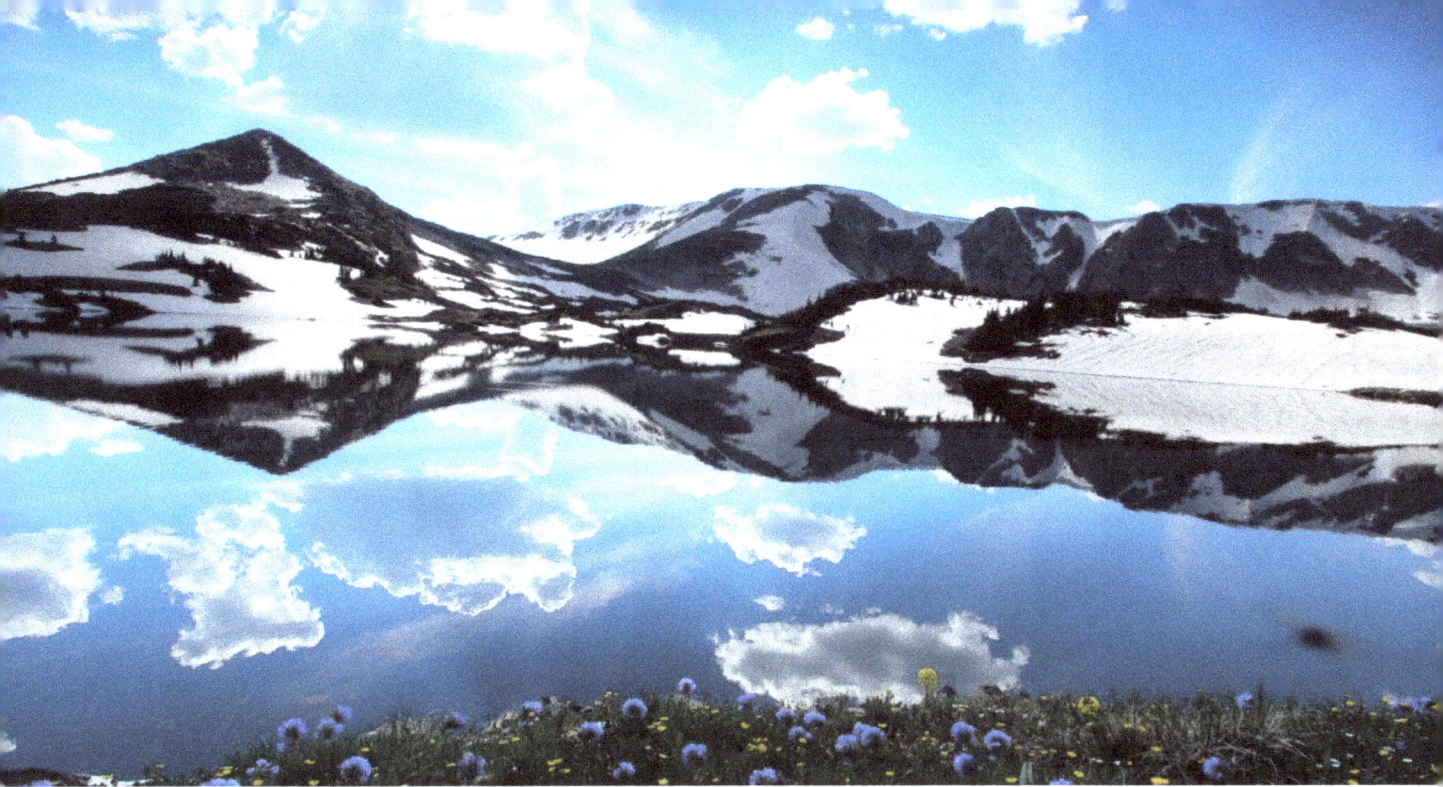

Introduction

"Invention, it must be humbly admitted, does not consist in creating out of a void, but out of chaos." ~ Mary Shelly

The inspiration for this book was a little surprising to me, as it happened partially in a bowling alley, and partially from watching a documentary on CTE's (chronic traumatic encephaly) in retired NFL players. The decision to join an amateur bowling league came at the same time the documentary aired. I'd had countless head injuries and concussions during my life and seeing my symptoms flare while trying to improve a game I hadn't played in decades reminded me not to let the indicators slide. There was a gap in proprioception whereby my brain sent no information about what my body was doing when I threw the ball. Seeing my body blank out like that was unnerving. I didn't want to wind up like those retired athletes!

Between the falls as a child, surgeries, martial arts, sports, and car accidents, I'd amassed dozens of traumas, many of which were to the head, throat, and brain. It took about forty years for the game-changing concussion later in life to make me aware of the cumulative effects of all the earlier injuries. I'd carried the symptoms over decades without realizing what a brain injury looks like. The signs weren't ignored because anyone in my family or circle of friends knew something should be done and I refused to seek care. The symptoms were ignored because they'd become a part of my growing up and couldn't be distinguished from any other discomfort you put behind you in spite of feeling not quite right.

Slowly, slowly, concussion after concussion, treatment after treatment, I began to gain a much-needed understanding of how a fall or bang on the head also impacts the brain and many other structures. I began to realize that a certain dysregulation can set in that creates susceptibility to additional injuries if left untreated. That's when I got serious about healing all the consequences of trauma wherever they may reside in my system. Curiosity turned into contemplation and investigations in a myriad of treatment modalities and trainings in therapeutic methods.

In spite of years of treatment, that day at the bowling alley showed that there was still work to do. At the same time something spontaneously lit up about how to share what contributed to my recovery process. Having already had three head injuries before I was six years-old, it makes me wonder what life might have been like if all my marbles were on board from the beginning. Watching that documentary helped connect the dots with the symptoms that could have been attributed to the brain trauma 40 years ago if anyone had known what to look for.

I remember reading decades ago that a surprisingly large percentage of death row inmates also had head injuries. Since some of the symptoms include increased aggression, poor decision-making, and poor impulse control, it made sense. The other populations that are vulnerable to brain injury are soccer, basketball, and hockey players, wrestlers, boxers

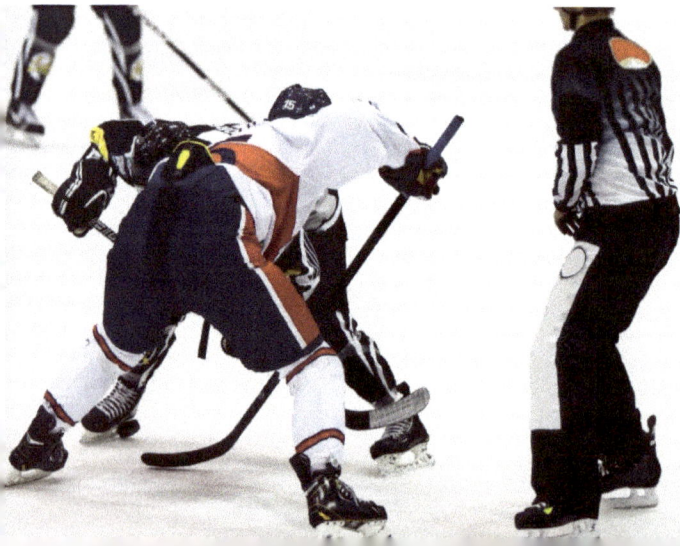

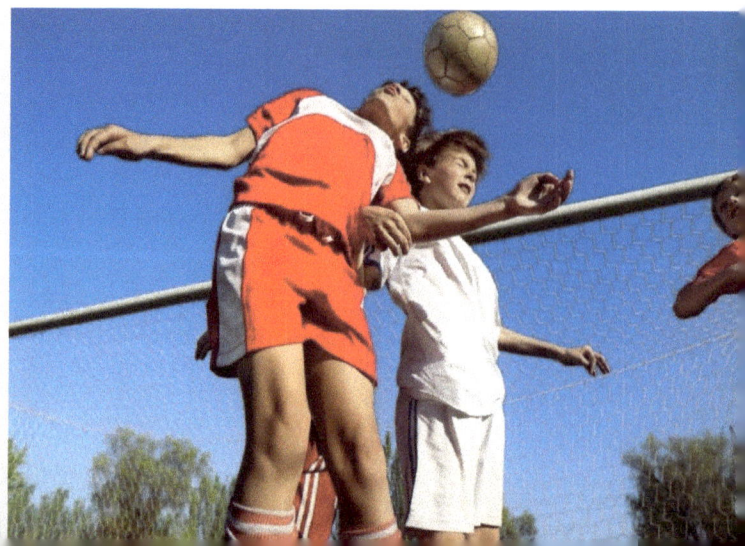

(called pugilistic dementia), martial artists, active combat soldiers and domestic abuse survivors. If it's so common, why hasn't anyone been talking about it? On the documentary one high school football player admitted that he didn't want to know about the dangers if they would mean that he couldn't play anymore.

In a sense, ignoring a head injury is like a form of gambling; like you'll take your chances if it means you can still do what you love. That may be the case for the younger players in general, as they still feel invincible and have a harder time seeing the future health consequences of their current actions when all they've known is vitality. The tide is finally changing for older athletes who've seen their friends go mad and commit suicide, or degenerate to a point of not being able to function. Although many professional athletes have had countless head and brain injuries, sometimes just one can alter a life forever.

I was surprised to find through Dr. Daniel Amen who showed through thousands of SPECT (Single Photon Emission Computerized Tomography) scans, that even a single event like a car accident can create brain changes that effect the personality, cognition, mood, affect, and other behaviors for life if not treated. He also has been working to show how these conditions that seem degenerative or permanent can greatly improve and probably heal using an anti-inflammatory diet, brain nutrition, and brain exercises. Since millions of head injuries happen every year, it has become a public health crisis.

The purpose of this book is to inform people how brain trauma happens, and how to recognize the symptoms; to let everyone know that effective treatment for the brain does exist, and that getting treated right away can make a huge difference. Understanding the dangers of contact sports, accidents, falls, and head injuries related to the brain could prevent unnecessary problems as we age. Unless this information is widespread among significant others who will notice changes in behavior and temperament, the physical symptoms might be more easily dismissed. Therefore, informing parents, teachers, coaches, medical staff, friends, therapists, and family members would do well to be informed and encourage patients or loved ones to not ignore the risks.

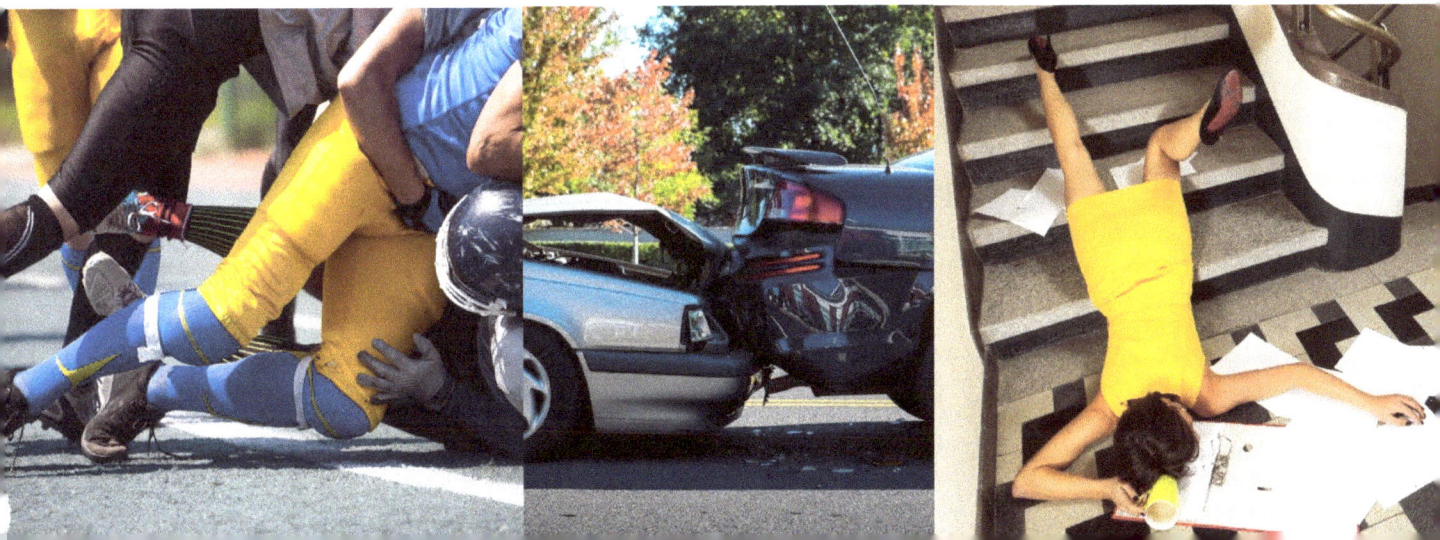

Children often would think nothing of a fall or injury unless there's a good deal of swelling and a parent sees that an emergency room visit is indicated. Otherwise, kids most likely don't even mention it while they're out playing unless it bleeds. I've had many clients come in and remember having fallen out of a window or off of a roof or tree without going to the doctor. An elderly client with scoliosis recalled falling onto a tiled fireplace without treating it and subsequently noticed the rearranging of her spine both in the kyphotic and scoliotic patterns that became problematic later on. Many times it may seem like the body is coping when it's really just compensating and running out of currency in its reserves.

Puberty and menopause bring on so many physiological and mood changes that it can be difficult to distinguish changes from injury perturbations or those from hormones and change of life issues. A restless, crying infant may have sustained cranial pressures during the birth process that often is in fact a trauma, particularly if forceps or a vacuum method was used. If the bones and membranes didn't balance in an optimal way, and while it may or may not produce an injury, a preventable dysregulation or discomfort could create issues that affect sleep, digestion, mood, and feeding.

In my lifetime being 'clumsy' or accident prone was never attributed to having had a head injury where having your bell rung could reorganize your body's ability to function in a coordinated way going forward. Writing this book will hopefully shine some light on a subject that's been in the dark for too long and that can in fact keep us in the darkness of our unconsciousness in ways that can be difficult to perceive because our perceiving mechanisms have been altered and diminished. It's such good news that now we can take another look at ADD, ADHD, depression or mood disorders, dyslexia, impulsive behavior, chronic headaches, and so many other symptoms that we'd otherwise take medication for or learn to live with.

Also, navigating the territories of musculo-skeletal reactions to head and brain trauma can be sketchy because it's so unfamiliar. What happens in the brain can have a global impact in the system. In fact, any injury can produce a global impact. Therefore, approaching the restoration process by including the entire system can and does produce more comprehensive, lasting results and may provide answers to why some issues remain chronic. It may also help to learn what makes injuries worse because I made a lot of mistakes either from being in denial, or through not understanding what I was up against.

Along the way I found it more useful to train in several of the modalities that were most helpful in my recovery, not only so I could use them on my own system when it flared up, but also to provide help to others who were trying to recover from injuries. I'm now inspired to discover the cause of flare-ups and eliminate them. I trust that there will be some useful information provided here for certain practitioners as well as patients as to what is available to treat the various aspects of traumatic brain injury, along with why it can be valuable to take action before cumulative insults to the system become debilitating.

It's pretty exciting to be able to include the results of the bowling inquiry in this text, as the writing and the bold move to join an amateur league will be simultaneous. The question now is, will conscious awareness have a tangible impact on what has fallen into the gravitational pull of a shadowy, tranced-in area and be able to pull it out again? At this late stage, will the exacerbated symptoms be able to yield to new or improved wiring like neuroplasticity research suggests? Can those improvements be reflected in a better body-brain connection that produces proper bowling form and flow amounting to better scores? We'll see. Whether physical, physiological, or metaphysical approaches prove to make the biggest difference, I trust the sharing of the journey will prove to be valuable for the reader.

Chapter 1

Living in a Fog

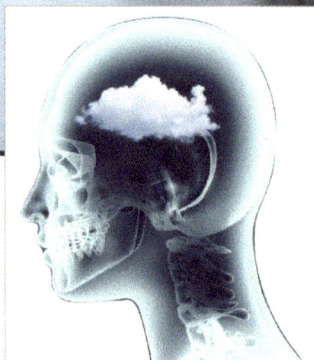

*"Consciousness does not create itself – it wells up from unknown depths.
In childhood it awakens gradually, and all through life it wakes each morning
out of the depths of sleep from an unconscious condition"*

– Carl Jung, (Collected Works, Vol. 11)

One of the conundrums about living in a brain fog is that it's often difficult to tell that you're in one. That's one of the reasons why writing this could be the fog horn in the distance that might help others who can relate to the journey; who might be able to notice the similarity in body and mind changes after an accident. Looking back, after being able to understand the symptoms more clearly, many issues that were present and unattributed to the early episodes could have been dissolved if my family had known what to expect and how to handle it. That being said, not much was known by anyone in those days beyond basic emergency care like stitches, pain medication, and the like.

Trauma tends to render the psyche into subconscious reflexive behaviors and perceptions, but awakened consciousness can see through the fog. For that reason this text will explore how consciousness can participate in the healing process. Viewing a condition or syndrome in terms of what happens to the consciousness or awareness of the person is fairly recent in rehabilitative settings. They're usually seen as separate in both causation and in treatment. Treatments for injuries are limited to the damage sustained in the tissues and bones; treatment for the psyche happens in the office of a psychologist or psychiatrist.

Neurologists may often prescribe something to enhance the firing of neurons, psychotherapists and psychiatrists may prescribe something to combat depression, but those meds don't heal the brain. The appearance of Somatic Experiencing, Hakomi, and Focusing in recent decades has started combining the idea that psychological issues can be released through where they connect and live in the body, as expressed by the sensations (not emotions) they create. Discharging trauma and reeducating the brain through sensation can access subconscious regions that will not respond as well to verbal or intellectual approaches, or to medication alone. These methods facilitate becoming a part of the sensory-motor feedback loop and being in direct communication with the brain using the brain's own language in the form of mechanoreceptors responsible for proprioception, and in the form of neurotransmitters responsible for temperament.

The prevalence of Alzheimer's disease in recent years has created an explosion of research into how and why the changes in the brain could generate such catastrophic health and personality disruptions. Some of these studies have yielded exciting results. Even schizophrenia has been seen to improve through modifying the microbiome. The discovery of the enteric nervous system has revolutionized the way we look at the brain and other systems. They're now seen as being a distributed, multi-directional hierarchy rather than a top-down organization. The brain can be profoundly affected by the presence or absence of certain bacteria and biochemicals in the gut as well as being influenced by the bones, heart, pancreas, lifestyle, emotions, and daily activities.

Now that it's able to be known that several areas of the body and brain are altered in a head injury, it just makes sense to also approach recovery as a multi-modal process. Rehabilitation should include reeducating the brain based upon the various regions that have been altered, reprogramming the senses, opening restricted fluids and energies, optimizing mobility of joints, fascia, and organs, correcting the compromised feedback from the musculoskeletal system wherever possible, as well as cultivating mindfulness and brain nutrition. This can not only help the brain to awaken out of a fog of cellular dysregulation, but can also enhance and support the entire process by employing the constituents of consciousness itself that is always awake on a certain level.

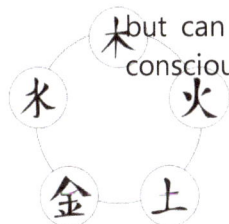

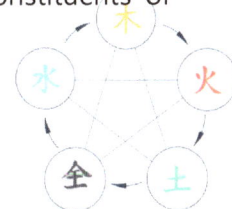

Following the Seeds on the Path

I believe that everyone is blessed with good fortune along the way, even and particularly in the midst of challenges. Looking back, I could see the progression of events that acted like a beacon in a sea of fog, directing the way to shore. Evolving out of studies in Special and Elementary Education, I was excited to discover the specialty area of Systems Intervention and Prevention in School Psychology. The premise of reorganizing the school system in order to avoid learning and behavior problems sounded enticing and potentially more effective than teaching to the test as a teacher. It also provided a perfect backdrop for what was about to take place in my life.

The college years were when my brain injury symptoms began to increase. I don't doubt that participating heavily in martial arts classes contributed to that fact. You get pretty fit in karate, but you also get pounded and injured on a regular basis. It was not cool to mention injuries or to complain. I did exactly what I now recommend not to do. I struggled to maintain a B+ average during undergrad years, because my brain was fading and a type of depression and overwhelm was growing. Dr. Wonderly didn't require a lot of reading for our grad classes, but he did require a lot of thinking and problem solving, several papers, and presentations.

A few of us signed up for this new program that studied the psychology of change and how to gently, without threat, intervene in a working system and create a change in a positive direction that is harmonious with what is already in place. My grad advisor not only planted seeds about a holistic approach to mental health, but he had also inspired a huge question mark about the nature of existence. Dr. Wonderly had stimulated an inquiry into who and what we are as human beings, as well as into what anything we perceive is. He jarred a type of awakening that started to sluff off a type of unconsciousness that I'd struggled with as a child to avoid but couldn't yet name. After he pointed out that humans basically functioned like Pavlov's dogs, he took things into another zone.

"What is this?" he'd ask, pointing to the object on the table in front of the classroom.
"A cup?" ventured one student.
"That's what we label it, but what *IS* it?"
"Something we drink out of?" another student offered.
"That's what we use it for, but what *IS* it?" he repeated.
"A piece of clay in a particular shape?" offered another brave soul.
"That's what it's made out of, but you're still not telling me what it *IS!*"

Silent stares filled the room as we waited in awe for him to fill the gaps in our dimly lit awareness. Where he took us on that existential ride was more exhilarating to me than everything we learned in all my undergrad years combined. He was evoking from us rather

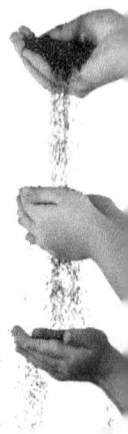

than data dumping into us, and something began to stir that hadn't been called forth in the past sixteen years of my education. He was stimulating was more than just intellect; he was also awakening a type of consciousness that I hadn't experienced before. It was different than the urge to lift out of the foggy nature of the brain dulled by trauma; it was more like an urge to awaken out of the fog socked in by life. I wanted to realize more fully what consciousness actually was and how it dove-tailed into the capacity for special abilities that I'd witnessed at martial arts tournaments, and that nearly every creature alive surpasses the human being in. I'd heard around this time that developing more sensitivity was related to diet, and that cumulative toxins could be dulling and unhealthy for the body.

Within a year of graduating I'd stopped eating beef and pork and began fasting once a week. Eating lighter was creating more of a desire to eat even less, so before and after the days of fasting I'd be drawn to eat just soups or salads. Life was moving so fast during college years - having gotten married and birthed a beautiful daughter while working as an intern and taking classes - that I pushed aside the inner struggles that were beginning to increase. I'd sustained many blows to the body, some to the head and neck during karate classes, and one during a black belt graduation test that was sufficient to rearrange my lower teeth. I was pretty fast, but not faster than everyone. The punch to the neck and throat was intentional. A sore loser during a match slugged me after I'd put my guard down and was walking back to the center of the ring to bow to her.

Post-concussive conundrum

I could swallow again the next day and although I was still able to sing, I do believe my pitch suffered after that. It didn't stop me from going to the dojo, as me and another student were teaching the class by then. A visit from an ex-sensei planted another seed after he told us that he'd begun to study with a martial arts Master. All of the martial artists who'd made impressive half-time demonstrations during the tournaments were either a high ranking black or red belt (beyond black), or a Master. I really loved that 76 year-old Master who performed a kata with the grace, flexibility, balance, and strength of someone half his age. Not that I wanted to break a board without touching it or blindfold myself and stop a sword an inch away from someone's bare skin. I didn't want the skills; I wanted to know how it was possible. I wanted to meet a martial arts Master.

Not long after graduation from grad school more brain injury symptoms became apparent. It was difficult to read more than a few paragraphs at a time and there was

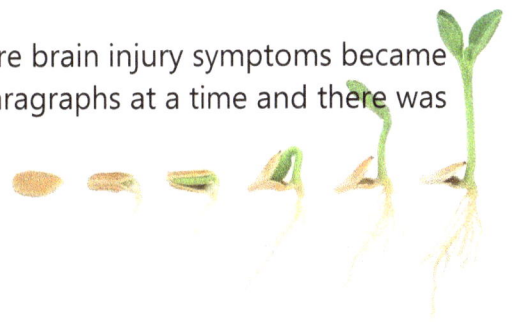

no guarantee that any of those words would register. I'd re-read them several times to get the gist, and only parts of simple magazine articles had a chance of being retained even briefly. These were symptoms someone 40 or 50 years older than me would experience. I felt at the time that it was brain fatigue from six years of college without taking a break and would soon self-correct but it didn't.

My family and I moved to Atlanta where I continued to work out in self-defense for a while before taking a position as a school psychologist. The children I assessed had complex emotional, behavioral, and neurological challenges that even a pediatric neurologist didn't have remedies for. My caseload was enormous, so I tried to at least get the children out of classes that were inappropriate for them, train the teachers, and make lists of specific exercises and activities to use in the classroom. My quest now included understanding the reason for the neurological deficits in these children if I could.

Serendipity takes hold

The dots began to connect themselves. Serendipity had led me to a person who was learning from a martial arts Master in New York City. Rather than describe the classes to me or let me observe, he insisted that I needed to experience them for myself. Since they were over 800 miles away, I had a big decision to make. I'd become one of those people who went through life on the surface as a part of a seemingly happy family, fully engaged in life, a career, hobbies, and as a wife and mother while being 80% numb inside. I say this only in looking back, because at the time, there were no words for what I was feeling because I wasn't feeling.

Decades later I discovered that flat affect could be a symptom of head injuries. At this point meeting a Master felt like my only lifeline so I grabbed onto it and moved to New York. I found a living situation that was life changing. My roommate introduced me to a spiritual Master and my first bodywork session. The session was in a modality I'd never heard of called Shiatsu. I was so impressed by its holistic nature I began studying and practicing Shiatsu to pay the bills and find ways to heal. Serendipity wasn't finished offering possibilities. The Dwa Shaan classes demanded everything. Nothing less than 200% effort was acceptable physically, energetically, and emotionally. No mental engagement was required or included, since what was being developed needed to come from another part of us.

I was a little surprised that we didn't very often get to spend time with the Master of the art, but he did drop in occasionally. There was a similarity between what he taught and what was taught in Aikido, in that the inner energetic development could be so profound that a mature practitioner could use the other person's energy to throw them off balance without using contact. Dwight stated at one point, "Before you can learn a self-defense method, you have to know the self you want to defend." Fertilizer was being added to the seeds. We worked every exercise in every class until it wasn't possible to move a muscle. I learned without a doubt at that time that there were energy reserves far beyond what anyone would imagine was possible, but who was this self I wanted to defend? What did that have to do with these painful exercises?

I got up from our exercises and fell down over and over again until I was unconscious and couldn't respond. That's a little ironic, isn't it – going unconscious in order to be able to be more conscious? Super counter-intuitive, but I had a lot of faith in the process, and held onto it until a stronger indication came to point me in a different direction. One of the goals in those classes was to work all the muscles so completely to open the body that it would relax every tension by intentionally creating maximum tension. We'd watch the body change shape as it opened, and the teacher took photos periodically so that we could see the difference. Tissues that were previously pulled into toward the core were released into external rotation.

A new kind of Zen stick

We learned that emotions and early experiences were stored in those muscles that had been contracting to hide or protect their unwanted expression. We knew that because after working so diligently to open everything everywhere, emotions began discharging fervently each week. We created a safe space outside of the gym for those times, as any emotion that arose in the gym was required to be put back into the exercises. There was a budding connection beginning to happen between the ability of the body to be energetically free, alive, and responsive and its ability to let go of stored experiences which were driving it toward numbing unconsciousness.

I couldn't tell if things were getting better or getting worse. I was so sore and spent after every class I could barely go up the subway stairs. This went on for two years with preparatory exercises until we finally got to the point where we were to attempt one punch. We repeated this one jab over and over and over for hours in the attempt to have it leave and land at the same time. Somehow we were trying to defy time and space and I loved the Zen koan of it all. The third year we were also given a series of movements that were similar to those in a kata, but we moved around the entire floor instead of in straight lines. The point was also not to throw techniques along the way, but to find from within how to effortlessly let the energy move us with no internal resistance.

It was like opposing gravity and other laws of physics while we danced in a flow that seemed to come from water and air instead of being earthbound. Because I'd seen and heard about so many remarkable feats by martial arts and later spiritual Masters, my mind was pretty open to almost anything being possible. Still, my jaw dropped a bit when the martial arts Master told me he'd killed a few attackers without touching them. He added that what we were practicing was none other than self-defense, not dance, not yoga, and that when you go to strike someone you had to be clear the intent was to have your full force behind it. It was up to them to decide whether or not to be hurt by the blow.

I could honestly say that I didn't really carry the intent to harm and didn't want to, although being able to defend myself sounded okay. There was a flaw in that theory to generate maximum tension in order to relax; some of those contractions didn't let go afterwards. I wasn't sure why. As much as I'd appreciated the Zen koan of trying to prepare the body to effortlessly transmit and receive energy and to perfect a timeless punch, in the end I realized that my path was one of 'do no harm'.

In the meantime I'd become a vegetarian and started meditating, but my body and mind continued on a downward spiral. While aligning with a deeper purpose was gratifying, my social life fell into the toilet and my mothering capacity went with it. I'd gotten hit in the head again in a paddle ball game requiring stitches, and sank into a deepening depression. Was it because we had to learn to fall to the floor during each martial arts class without protecting ourselves? Possibly. Was it because I got hit so hard with the metal edge of a paddle that my forehead opened up? Maybe that additional trauma took things over the edge.

India drops into me

All the rapid-fire changes had been too much to understand, integrate, and be with comfortably. I went to India for answers to visit the teacher in the book I'd read. I heard so many stories of miracles around him that I believed he was a true Master because his reach was beyond time and space and felt multi-dimensional. His presence felt vast and limitless and he saw things clearly. The seeds being dropped along the way opened the next opportunity to further the quest and questions around consciousness, healing, and the nature of life. Bhagwan recommended a few workshops for me which proved to open new doors in consciousness. At the end of the one called, 'Centering' an experience opened that revealed the difference between awareness and attention. There was definitely a type of consciousness beyond the body that could be aware and awake and perceiving 360° without effort. It was like having eyes in the back of my head. Although that state of awareness didn't remain past that day, we were encouraged to maintain that fire of being aware throughout daily activities and not allow the mind to fall back into a dull trance-like sleepy place.

One famous Zen story I heard Bhagwan tell one day further sealed the commitment. The story ends with the Master Nan-in asking his student, *"Then tell me, did you place your umbrella on the right or left side of your shoes?"*

The student replied, "I've no idea, Master."

"Zen Buddhism is the art of total consciousness of what we do," said Nan-in. "The lack of attention to the smallest details can completely destroy a man's life"

I could wholeheartedly agree that I'd been in such a fog that I'd not attended to the details of my life in a consistent way and much chaos had ensued as a result. I hadn't followed reason generally, but usually something in front of me that was compelling at the time. The third experience Bhagwan suggested for me was a Samadhi tank. In this sensory deprivation tank filled with a saline solution closely matching that of the waters in the womb, I floated out of depression and into a field of sparkling bliss for three days. What a contrast to all those strenuous approaches to martial arts!

Excited about being in his Buddha field while continuing these explorations in consciousness, I sold everything I owned and moved to India with my daughter. I gave Shiatsu sessions to visitors, trained in Breath Therapy or Rebirthing, taught the guards martial arts, sang in a celebration band, and participated in many other activities in the community for almost two years. If I sang flat, nobody cared. The Rebirthing sessions were meant to build so much energy in the system through the breath, that held imprints or impressions would lift out on a sea of prana. Every session was absolute bliss. So much so that I thought I'd never need another therapeutic process in my life, but my emotions were still all over the place.

India was over the top for my daughter who later left to live with her father. It proved to be challenging for others as well, as one of our guards and martial arts students had a brain aneurysm and perished. I couldn't explain why, but during the period of his coma and subsequent departure from his body, my heart opened. All those years of being numb inside shifted in a couple of days. Was it Grace, having a deeper connection with the student than we realized? Was it the sublime nature of his transition or the magic of the Buddha field? Probably all of the above. For weeks after that a profound stillness permeated my being. There was such peace and utter contentment that all of me had been captured by it.

No interests or concerns arose; no distractions or desires could compete with this state of rest. I don't know that there were any thoughts to speak of, and I mostly didn't speak at all, but sat quietly for hours on end. The numbness was thawing as the Heart of hearts began to come alive. It was just a tiny glimpse of the realization that the Kingdom of Heaven really *IS* within.

The body sinks as the spirit soars

I returned back to the U.S. more than a year later, full of energy on one level, but physically weaker than I'd ever been in my life. My body was unable to digest more than soup. I'd had good health for the most part while in India, with the exception of a bout with Giardia, amoebas, and dengue fever. There was also a mystery disease that I never could identify but received a mystery medicine for from an Indian doctor who said he was an eye doctor, but hey – when you're that sick you'll try anything. The main thing is that it worked.

There was also a strange period where my urine was the color of coca cola that I assumed was related to my liver, but didn't get it tested since it didn't last and didn't slow me down. However, the transition back to the West was a rough one. Within five years I'd gone from being the most fit I've ever been in my life to the weakest and most unhealthy I'd ever been. Was it related to the doses of Flagyl I'd taken for the buggies in my belly? I don't doubt that it had a strong effect. I'd also noticed that my mind with its mental acuity was fading. While being submerged in a quest for greater consciousness, my body and intellect were ironically in peril. I developed allergies and food intolerances, almost zero digestive powers, mood swings, depression, suicidal tendencies, and a big time mental fog. My blood sugar and blood pressure were so low that I was passing out, my joints wouldn't stay in place which created ankle sprains, a hyper-mobile spine, chronic muscle spasms, inflammation, and eventually a bulging disc.

I hadn't had a good night's sleep in years. I'd gotten my tubes tied in India and although the doctors couldn't find anything, I couldn't walk fast for almost a year without a strange pull in my groin. I went to an acupuncturist who practiced iridology and she gasped when she looked into my eyes. "You have ball pockets in your intestines like someone much older would have. You stop eating right now, go on a fast for a week and cleanse your system," she said. She also gave me herbs for my kidneys as well to help balance my hormones. I began taking probiotics daily. I didn't get better, but the stuff that came out of my intestines was scary. Was the missing link still my brain injuries? Why didn't she see them in my eyes?

Somehow, paradoxically, efforts to increase in consciousness had cost me a fundamental mental alertness and decision-making capacity. I couldn't help but wonder if I was going to wind up too dim-witted to be able to understand what was happening, but was so enthralled by the realms of experiencing that were so much more vibrant, I just kept following where it led, but hopefully not to early-onset dementia in the name of a spiritual awakening or the like. If only I could have processed information effectively I could have

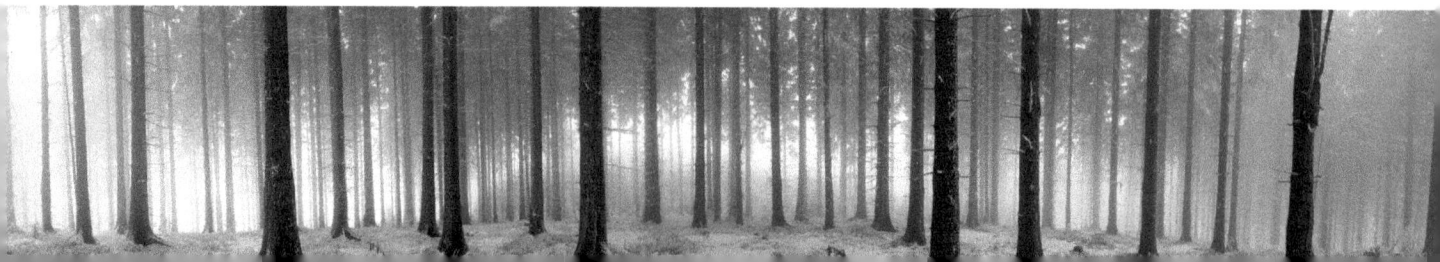

asked the right questions. Instead I landed in a different type of fog. I loved the street life in Manhattan, as it reminded me of the outdoor culture that was so vibrant in India, but the day I went for a walk and blew black soot out of my nose I decided to leave. Soon I moved to the West Coast and continued studying the body, the subconscious mind, energy fields, and various forms of manual medicine. I now needed to heal body and brain, but I also wanted to understand it. For that I also needed to get my mind back. I set my sights on a shift in my career track and on anything that might restore normal functioning in my now incredibly delicate system.

Landing in California after living in New York and India was a breath of fresh air, literally! I was amazed by the fragrance in the flowers and the flavor in the fresh produce, as well as the beauty in the sprawling nature of every kind, and the creatively landscaped neighborhoods. In the search for work I was hired by an orthopedic, sports, and physical therapy clinic where I was able to both learn about injuries and to help treat them. My own body was still pretty weak but I think I hid it pretty well. My boss was helpful in resetting my then hyper-mobile spine, sacrum, and pelvis, yet the chronic spasms, pain, and inflammation persisted.

The years in Dwa Shaan had prepared me for a mindset whereby I just knew that the body was capable of so much more than we realized. We'd learned to put the energy of the pain into the exercise and keep going, so I redirected that energy into doing my job. Many days I hopped up and down the stairs because I couldn't put weight on one leg, and I finally avoided sitting down as it compressed the injured disc. I strapped some ice to my back with a back brace and pushed on. While treating patients there using heat, ice, phonophoresis, traction, and massage, the issue of acute versus chronic conditions was at the forefront of my curiosity. There were several falls, car accidents, repetitive strains, and sports injuries each week. After my portion of the treatment, the physical therapists would come in and assess the patient, do various manipulations, and send them to the gym for exercises.

Most patients came three times a week until they were better, or until their insurance benefits ran out. It was great to see patients so regularly and have a chance to observe their process. It was fascinating to see in this context as well that some people seemed to continue injuring themselves. Before fully healing from one car accident they'd have another one, or barely a few weeks after a carpenter healed a repetitive strain injury, he'd have a fall. Chronic and repeat injuries became more and more intriguing. For the complex injuries received due to auto accidents, I started asking, "Where were you sitting in the car when the accident happened? Where was the car hit?" I'd compare that information with where their

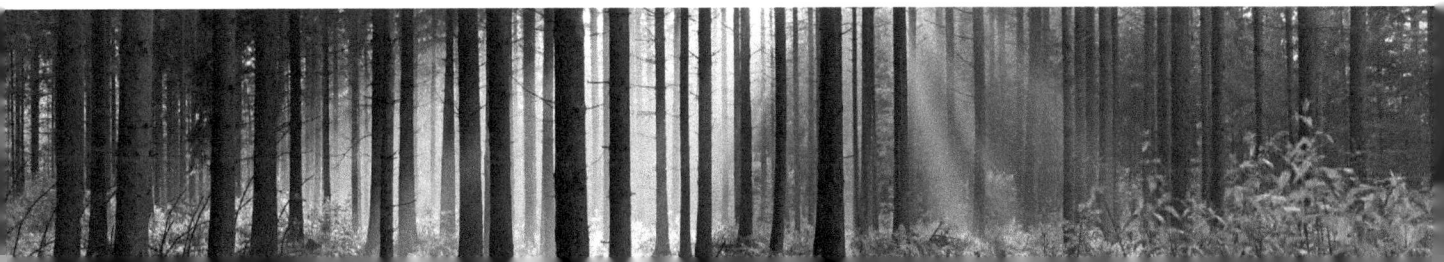

symptoms were and see if a pattern was emerging related to where undissipated forces were landing in their system. My palpation skills weren't developed enough at that time to make use of the information.

I'd taken a sports injury class with an orthopedic surgeon around that time who explained that there was a cycle to the healing process, and if another pain signal is instigated while the body is trying to shift to the repair and remodel stage, it will revert back to the injury stage and regenerate earlier inflammation and guarding. Inflammation, I learned recently, is part of the healing process and is only a problem if it becomes chronic. Almost everyone, including myself, began to over-exert themselves as soon as they started to feel better, exacerbating the symptoms and reverting to earlier phases of the healing process. It's particularly misleading if pain medication is muddying the waters of perception and the injury doesn't actually feel as good as you think it does.

I was beginning to wonder if we couldn't see the forest for the trees. It seemed like the whole rehabilitation system was designed to make the area that was feeling the most pain feel better instead of considering all of the contributing factors. The body also did its best to compensate and substitute in ways that enabled functioning to continue without loading the weakened area. Becoming convinced of the intelligence of the body and the specificity of its resources, adaptability, and resiliency, I had to wonder what could stimulate the release of chronic injury patterns. Did it hold on only in absence of accurate messaging, or due to the fact that additional injury was being interpreted by the system?

I reflected on some of Dr. Wonderly's discourses on systems intervention. The body was, after all, a very intricate system that in its own way was making decisions in the direction of self-preservation every minute of the day. To illustrate what was needed for real change to happen, Dr. Wonderly drew an image on the board of a network of fibers tied in to the same fabric or web. He helped us to understand that trying to remove one strand tied into that network wouldn't work unless the other related strands were also addressed. The same applied to memories or gestalts in the psyche or nervous system. If there was an emotional component, or an association with the status quo that symbolized security, identity, or safety, there would be resistance to change. It seems the same held true for the body.

The elephant in the room

I don't remember hearing about a concussion as being part of the problem, even though many of the car accidents and falls patients described must have included one. There were pedestrians getting hit by cars, ski accidents, whiplash injuries, falls from ladders, and stress fractures of the spine that seemed like there must have been some trauma to the head, but it was never mentioned and never included in the treatment protocol. Was that part of the elephant in the room of the condition called 'chronic'? A wise man once said that if even the tail of the elephant is still in the room, the entire elephant can be pulled back in. I do remember the mention of coup/contrecoup - with the brain hitting both the front and back of the skull - as being part of most any whiplash, but there was a gaping hole in knowing what to do about it. It wasn't within the scope of practice of physical therapy in those days. How many people continued in their lives while experiencing aches and pains, pushing through with pain meds? I'd done it my entire life. It made me pretty eager to learn more about the kingpin of the recovery process for each person and hopefully get to the bottom of my own hot mess.

Over time we'd heard of various professionals at the top of their field in manual therapy and the head of the clinic was open to inviting them for an in-service for the staff. One of the presenters described how muscles around an injury are sent inhibitory signals from the brain so that they would weaken and the person was less inclined to do much while the area is restoring itself. The presenter who peaked my interest the most was Dr. Tom Hanna. He demonstrated the neurophysiological principles behind his techniques that he claimed could shift even the most long-standing patterns in a short period of time. That was certainly proven in my case.

He'd called his approach the 'missing link' in resetting muscle tension, pain, and imbalances. Hanna Somatic Education was based in Feldenkrais work which had evolved as Awareness through Movement and had a long-standing reputation for 'miracle' healings. Hanna Somatics made the changes through informing the brain of the body's current status by sending and receiving proprioceptive information via their receptors to and from the brain. Using a few specific, gradual, eccentric contractions along my spine made my body felt better in fifteen minutes than it had in over four years.

It sounded like he'd applied the same theory to the body that Dr. Wonderly applied to the psyche, in that muscles were tied into a web of simultaneous firing during any given activity, and releasing one muscle with the most discomfort wouldn't release the entire pattern. In fact, he proposed just the opposite – that by not including the entirety of the body's web of engagement through movement sequences that called for conscious, unified participation, the pattern would most likely return. That concept would be the same as the tail of the elephant.

It not only made a lot of sense, but the proof was also in the pudding when my back changed enormously in just a few minutes. At that time I'd been in pain and in a back brace for nearly four years, unable to stand, sit, or lie down without pain. Dr. Hanna had me repeat one movement a few times that incorporated all of the extensors in my body, and, "Poof!" like a feat of magic the spasms vanished. My amazement and appreciation turned into a

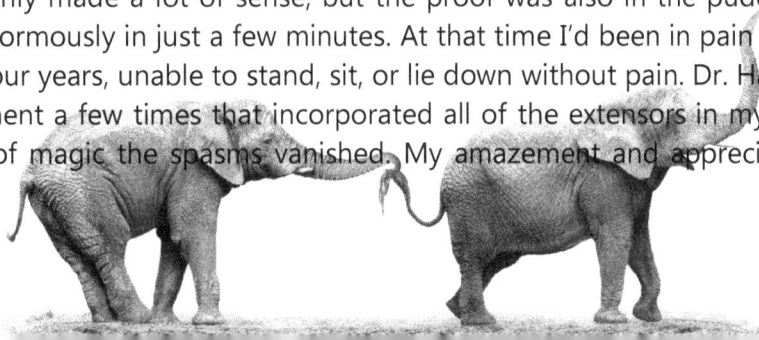

passion to learn more about the mechanisms behind that movement; I wanted to understand the principles behind why it worked. The other intriguing aspect of this demonstration was how confident Dr. Hanna was that it would work in every instance. Not a hint of this, "Individual results may vary" disclaimer was expressed by him.

I was convinced that the decisions made by the body had a reason, even if at some point that decision had become counter-productive. If Tom Hanna had the answer to this phenomena – and he appeared to – then I needed to be wherever he was going to be. Studying Hanna Somatic Education was my first in a long series of trainings about how the body can respond to new input regarding a dysfunction or imbalance and create the appropriate changes of its own accord. Tom had a theme running around 'the myth of aging' and the ways that the system could remain young and responsive if it could remain self-aware.

If the reports of the 100 year-old marathon runner, the 99-year old who graduated college after 70 years, the 106 year-old who zip lined on his birthday, and the 104 year-old Japanese doctor who goes to work every day aren't inspiration about the possibilities, I don't know who is. They each had goals and the motivation to achieve them. So whatever the research says about aging is not set in stone. Gladys Burrill, one of the oldest women to complete a marathon at 92 years old, walks up to 50 miles a week and reports that she never gets sore, even after a race. There must be a physiology in her worth studying.

During Hanna's training we learned about an occurrence he called, "sensory motor amnesia", whereby an area of the system has gone numb and is 'offline' or unable to give and receive new information to the brain. Without this link-up, other muscles may substitute or compensate for the fibers that are in the dead zone, eventually themselves becoming strained from overworking. Flexibility and dexterity are also lost because the integrated communication and delivery systems have lost a portion of their network. The purpose of the techniques and the movements in Hanna Somatics are to wake up those dormant fibers so they can reconnect with and inform the brain of the default patterns of imbalance that have arisen, and replace them with the original. After applying the neuromuscular reeducation methods during the training, I had an experience of being pain-free after one month.

It was such a glorious moment I stood still for few minutes to let it sink in; just to appreciate the sensation of normalcy and coherence. It showed me that improvement was not only possible, it was on the way. Unfortunately, there were as many movements that caused a flare-up as there were that greatly reduced it. It gradually became clear which ones my system could tolerate and improve with and which ones to avoid. Each activity in front of me required the same discernment during the healing process in order to not give pain signals to the brain and start the repair process all over again.

I began a delicate rehabilitation process that included water exercises, the Stairmaster, racquetball, and dance for aerobic conditioning, including Hanna Somatics for reeducation. Yoga wasn't acceptable to my body, nor were movements requiring extremes in rotation of the spine. At that point, even cold water could cause a spasm. My system was still quite vulnerable, but was going through the day with less and less pain. There was still a lot to learn Next on the agenda was to get stronger and understand how to prompt my system to consistently retain the changes to my low back and sacrum. I only learned later that a key component of the injuries being able to become chronic in my system at such a young age was the gut. Missing that component and the brain treatment component meant it took by body the longest time to heal. I'd say in about seven years my body was back to normal in the physical and physiological sense, but the cognitive issues would take even longer.

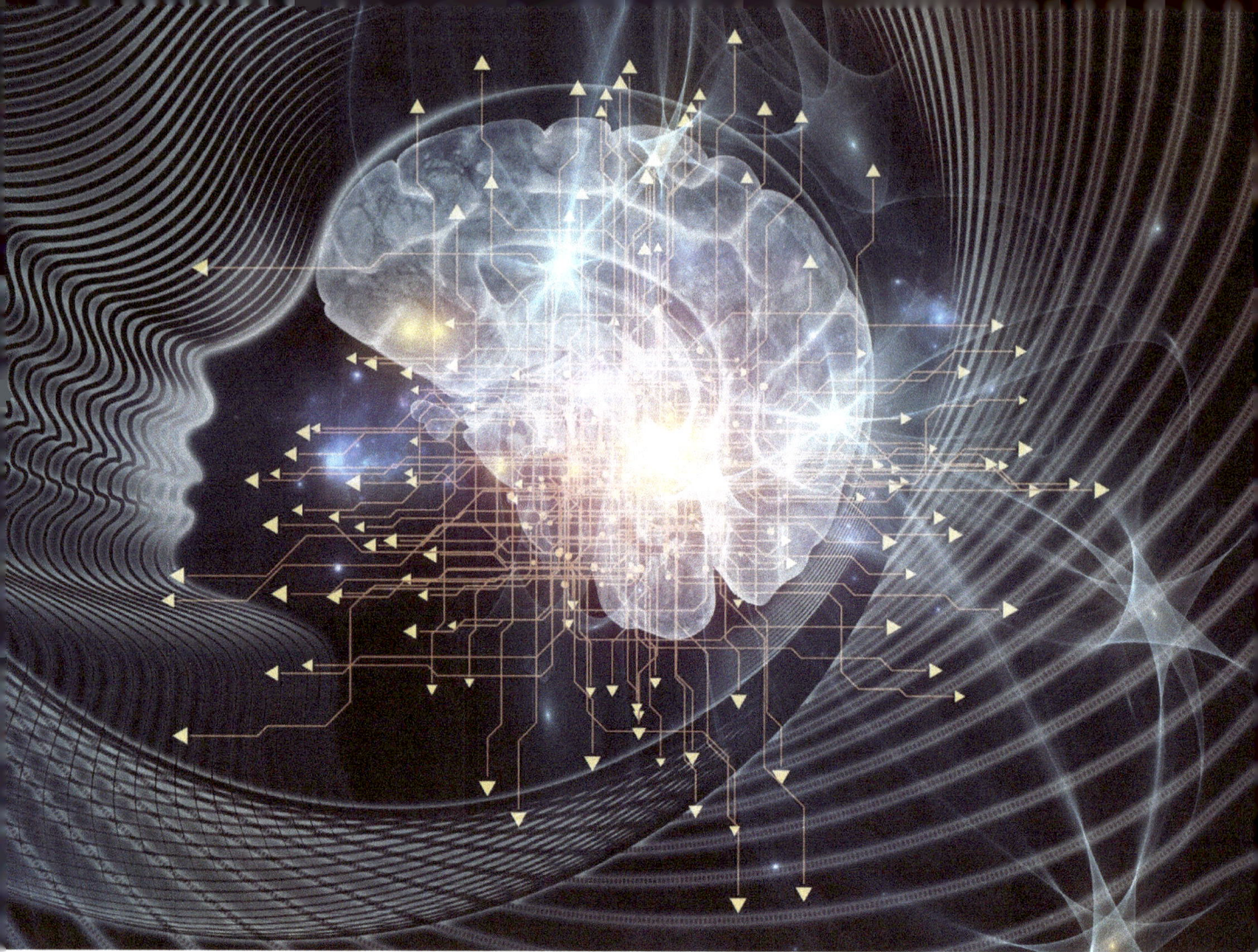

Chapter 2

The Inner Workings of Injuries

"Blows received by the cranium, after being conveyed to these poles, are dispersed thence in every direction to all its substances; and indeed in a most regular manner, according to every particular form, so that no injury to the form need be feared. Whatever flows or runs in accordance with the form never injures or violates the mass. But if anything runs counter to this form or in a different direction, then it causes an injury."

~ Emmanuel Swedenborg, (The Brain, Vol. 1, 1882)

Key components of injuries that are noteworthy here is that they can exist as lesions within multiple systems simultaneously, and that they rewire the brain, even if the injury didn't originate in the brain. They can also reach across time with different manifestations since all injuries exist within a web or network that can produce an effect in a variety of systems. For example, a brain injury can express in the shoulder one month, as dyslexia a few months later, in the belly as indigestion or nausea during another phase, and along the spine at still another point. That being the case, it may help to address the area of manifestation, but treat the source.

Sensory-motor amnesia was not only happening with my muscles at the bowling alley many years later, but there was also a 'blank-out' when the brain and body were on an inaccessible auto-pilot. The eyes were seeing, and the body was moving, but it was like in a dream. It was like a blind spot in the brain that wasn't sending sensory information about my right side, but just at the point where the ball was to be released. How fascinating and inspiring that was! I felt enormously lucky to be able to see it with the awareness that had become awakened in India. What a mess I was before! The shock that accompanied that repeated inability to gather all the parts back online generated the motivation to see it through to further healing and regaining of fuller body/brain consciousness.

The infamous list of mishaps

Let's go back and retrace some of the steps and missteps that led to the neural confusion that took almost a lifetime to recognize, investigate, and eventually overcome.

1. Fall down a full flight of 15 stairs at 1 year old
2. Hot water pours from a pan and burns my left arm
3. Iron burns my left hand – now I can see which side is left
4. Umbilical hernia surgery 2 years old
5. Blunt trauma - Stitches in my right forehead at 3 years old
6. Fall down the stairs onto my face again at 5 years old
7. Surgery for nasal ulcer at 6 years old
8. Tonsillectomy at 9 years old
9. Sprained left ankle 12 years old
10. Braces at 14 years old
11. Fighting in karate from 19 years old for 10 years
12. Throat injury at 23 years old
13. Jaw injury 24 years old
14. Fell through a hole in the floor, caught by my ribs and elbows 26 years
15. Blunt trauma -Stitches in my left forehead at 28 years old
16. Repeated falls in Dwa Shaan 27 – 29 years old

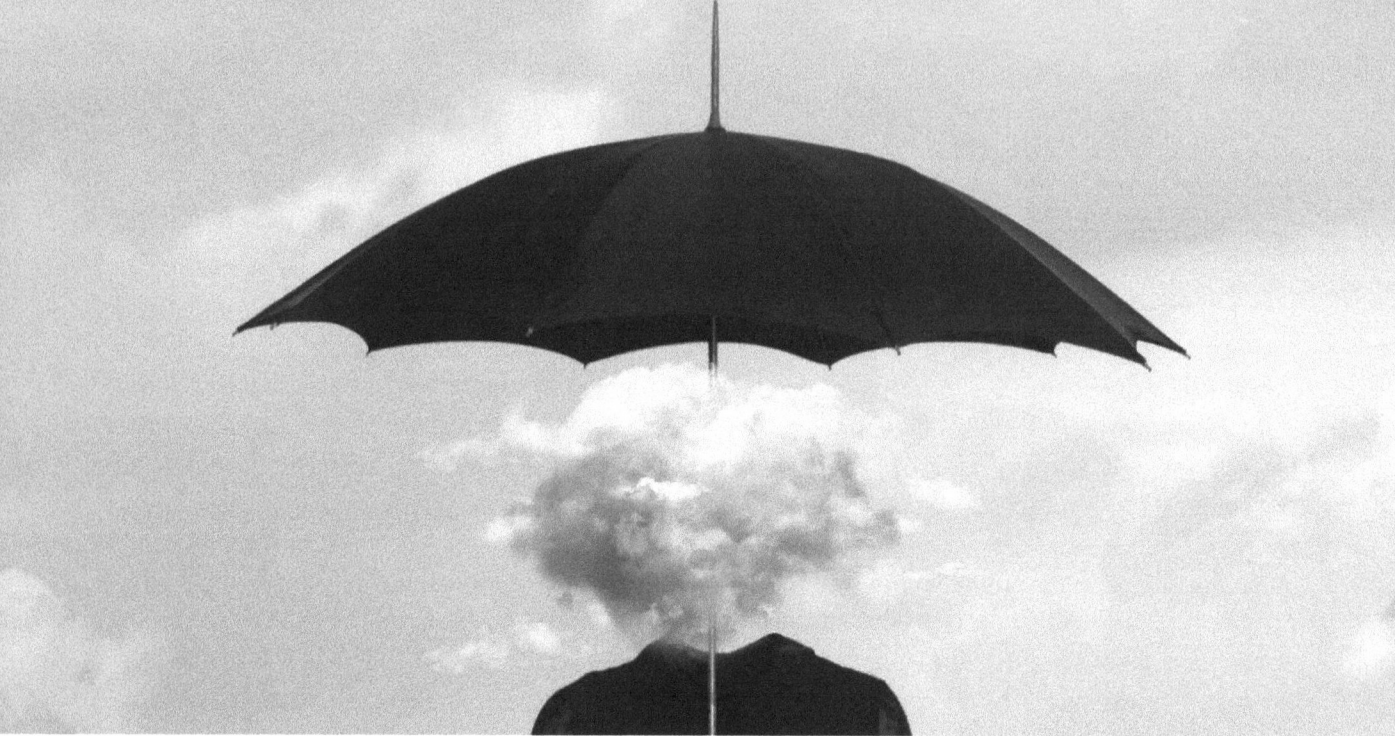

17. Tubal ligation 31 years old
18. Disc injury at 33 years old
19. Racquetball in the eye – post traumatic iritis 38 years old
20. Sprained right ankle 41 years old
21. Rear-end Whiplash 44 years old (coup contrecoup)
22. Broadside whiplash 45 years old
23. Sprained right ankle 46 years old
24. Failed drop table technique causing face pain 46 years old
25. Lost consciousness, fall on cement (concussion) 47 years old
26. Stone throw from 50 ft. up lands on my forehead 47 years old
27. Sprained right ankle 48 years old
28. Glass shower door falls on my forehead 48 years old
29. Broadside head injury 49 years old
30. Head bump on beam with slip & fall on deck 52 years old
31. About a dozen head bangs on doors, drawers, trees, low arbors
32. Slip & fall on a wet deck
33. About 5 different head bangs with items falling on head from upper shelves
34. Frozen shoulder right side
35. Seat belt injury/face with airbag injury 58 years old
36. Sprained right ankle 60 years old; Sprained left ankle 62 years old
37. Vacuum cleaner falls off hook onto right occiput 64 years old
38. Flower pot full of dirt falls off shelf onto left occiput 64 years old
39. Braces 66 years old
40. Head scrape 67 years old

41. Frozen shoulder left side
42. Head scrape 68 years old
43. Racquetball in the same eye 68 years old
44. Sprained left ankle 68 years old
45. Basketball to the head 68 years old

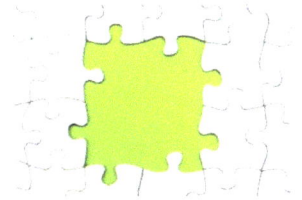

Brain changes following knee surgery

The first sixteen injuries in my life and countless falls and blows in martial arts seemed to be absorbed and processed fairly well by my system. Only afterwards the clumsiness, spatial disorientation, eye sensitivity, stiffness in my neck, memory issues, moodiness and depression landed as being attributable to those early traumas. Initially, spraining my ankle in a junior high gymnastics class didn't seem like a big deal, but it's been recently shown that the proprioceptors in the knee and ankle change the brain. The feedforward process from the brain to the joint is altered, creating impairments in the step, jump, and landing process of that leg. Researchers also observed change in cortical excitability involving inhibitory signals that could induce increased stiffness in the knee or increased laxity in the ankle (Pietrosimone et al, 2012).

A post-surgical study 16 months after the reconstruction of the ACL showed an unexpected reorganization of the brain. There was increased activation of the contralateral motor cortex, lingual gyrus, and ipsilateral secondary somatosensory cortex, with diminished activation in the ipsilateral motor cortex and cerebellum compared to healthy controls. The results were interpreted as this reorganization leading to a more visual- motor rather than sensory-motor reliance for movement of the reconstructed knee. In my mind that could mean it would be advisable to literally 'watch your step' when confronted with uneven surfaces or stairs rather than relying on the feel of the surface producing clear enough information to retain balance.

In addition, scar tissue may not be as dynamically active in responding to or accurately transmitting proprioceptive stimuli while also altering the tissue field's ability to yield to incumbent forces. Certain levels of tension and gathered forces that have not been evenly distributed or effectively discharged may generate additional alterations in posture, in gait, in coordination and dexterity, and in strength. There can also be changes in fluid dynamics resulting in blood pressure changes, lymphatic stagnation, or reduction in the flow in life force through the cerebral spinal fluid. Forces can accumulate that diminish organ and gland function and metabolic processes in general, either through fascial restrictions or biochemical changes related to stress, hypervigilance, or faulty messaging. All of this is to say that unresolved injuries can wreak havoc down the road and the resulting symptoms may not immediately be attributed to these earlier events What might the brain do to compensate after multiple injuries with corrective surgical interventions?

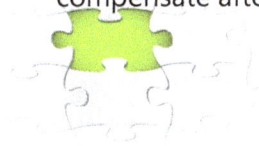

How much is the brain's organization further compromised when a joint has been resurfaced or replaced? What additional rehabilitation processes could be included when those realizations become widespread in treatment facilities? Hopefully brain changes and sensory-motor deficits will be taken into account in assessment and exercise prescriptions in the near future. Joints are warehouses full of proprioceptive input via the golgi tendon and ligament receptors, joint capsule, and skin that inform the brain of joint position. It makes a lot of sense that alterations in these structures can and will alter the accuracy of the information being provided, and therefore compromise the accuracy of the response from the brain based upon how it can assess the situation.

Wikstrom and Brown noted a cascade of joint changes after an ankle sprain that would dysregulate reflexes and create cortical remapping with sensorimotor reorganization that alters the brain's perception of the joint. Barral and Croibier also report that, *"During trauma, the mechanoreceptors are subjected to rough treatment. They react to strong mechanical forces by 'disinforming' local, regional, or central nerve centers. They either under-estimate or over-estimate the mechanical stimuli received. This proprioceptive 'disinformation' causes inappropriate muscular reactions which endanger the patient's general equilibrium, and (result in) leg or ankle sprains due to poor contraction or muscular coordination."* (Trauma - An Osteopathic Approach, 1997)

Biomechanical adaptations to injury and adhesions

The body continues to make subtle adaptations with each incident. Here's more of what's really happening underneath the skin while the mending is being supported in these traditional ways. Tissue fields are impacted by the initial trauma, surgical interventions as well as subsequent scarring. At the molecular level, there is constant cross-talk between the fascia, surrounding tissues, and their respective physiology. Zugel, Maganaris, et al, found that, *"All factors influencing cell or ECM (extra-cellular matrix) behavior can result in changes in the structure and homeostasis of tissues and organs. The ECM also works as a molecular store, catching and releasing biologically active molecules to help regulate tissue and organ function, growth, and regeneration."* (Journal of Sports Medicine, 2018)

In this regard, the researchers noticed that these molecules stored in the matrix can be released and activated during mechanical stressors, exercise, hormonal changes, and aging. Age-related alterations in fascial tissues include densification of loose connective tissue and fibrous collagen bundles, which often contribute to *"reductions in range of motion and force... and chronic, low-grade inflammation."* Since fascia also transmits force, modifications in that matrix due to adhesions, load shifting due to pain, or mal-alignment could also influence muscle mechanics which consequently effect strength, coordination, and balance. Even without a fall aging begins to sound like it's an injury unto itself but not an inescapable

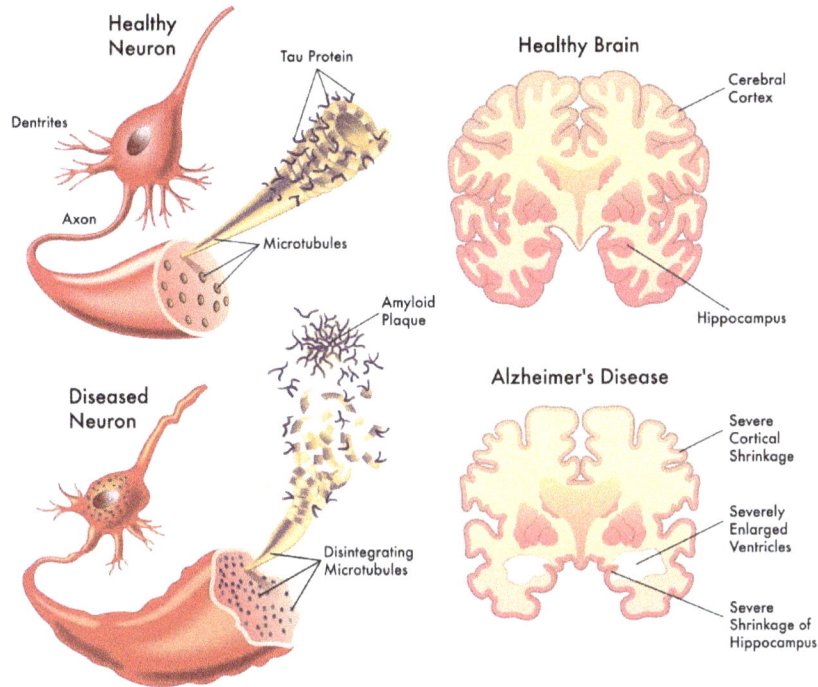

Healthy Neuron — Dentrites, Axon, Tau Protein, Microtubules

Diseased Neuron — Disintegrating Microtubules, Amyloid Plaque

Healthy Brain — Cerebral Cortex, Hippocampus

Alzheimer's Disease — Severe Cortical Shrinkage, Severely Enlarged Ventricles, Severe Shrinkage of Hippocampus

prognosis if steps are taken to unwind the 'life story' buried in the fascia and its constituents.

Luigi Stecco describes what happens when fascia distorts, *"If the soft tissues surrounding a joint do not stretch according to physiological lines, then the receptors embedded in these tissues signal the dysfunction as pain. Any therapeutic intervention therefore, is not to be focused at the site of pain or the center of perception as they are mere consequences of the dysfunction."* Zugel's researchers also discovered that some substances released during an injury (including overuse) *"promote immune cell proliferation in an acute phase including macrophages, cytokines, bradykinin, substance P, and proteases sensitizing nociceptive afferents."*

When in the system for an extended period of time, which can easily happen if the injury is misunderstood or underplayed, these substances can become toxic. The toxicity further stimulates immune responses and creates more tissue damage, increased adhesions, and fibrosis, especially near joints. It's been reported that having numerous closed head injuries could create structural changes in brain tissue, some of which have to do with shrinkage in various nuclei, inflammation, S100B or tau protein build up (traumatic brain injury marker), scar tissue, and stretching or rupture of axons rupture in the white matter. An important feature to remember is that although damage is taking place, we can remain unaware of it because there are also compensations that allow us to function for quite a while until inner adaptability or resources become limited. Similar to cancer and other conditions that can take years to develop to the point where the symptoms reach the surface, brain injuries are able to remain within a manageable spectrum until they pass a certain threshold.

Biochemical changes following trauma

Dr. Thomas McAllister, in his paper on *"Neurobiological consequences of traumatic brain injury,"* makes distinctions between a closed and penetrating brain injury whereby an object penetrates the brain. This text will only cover closed head and brain injuries that involve both concussive and sub-concussive traumas. McAllister points out that both the mechanical perturbations of the axons and of the cells can create an influx of extracellular calcium ions that then instigate reactions inside the cell leading to cytotoxic results and cell death, which can happen days or even weeks later.

In addition, cysteine proteases are set in motion, one set of which leads to decreased energy due to the apoptosis (cell death) process that then triggers inflammation. The other set (calpains substrates) causes a *"disruption of cell transport, and the destruction of cyto-architecture and cell membrane elements"* that also leads to death of the cell. (Dialogues in Clinical Neuroscience, Sept. 2011) Excessive amounts of excitatory neurotransmitters are released during trauma. For example, glutamate and excitatory amino acids in areas like the hippocampus and prefrontal cortex where they're found in higher amounts and where damage is often observed in brain injuries, likely explaining consequent memory and cognitive issues.

Neuropathologist, Ann McKee noticed shrinkage and atrophy in the prefrontal cortex, hippocampus, amygdala, and other areas associated with learning, memory, judgment, and emotional control in the brains of deceased NFL players. Dr. McKee estimated than on average an NFL lineman receives about 1200 sub-concussive hits in a single season, and that these hits create the same traumatic injury but with fewer symptoms. The cumulative effect though, after just a few years of playing the game is catastrophic. In addition, numerous players receive knee and ankle injuries that include surgical interventions. Increased tissue density and fascial restrictions will further alter signaling throughout the matrix and reduce the range and efficiency of movement.

The good news is, that since the lawsuits and publicity emerged about the dangers of concussions in the NFL, several new helmets have been produced that can sense rates of acceleration upon impact, and a couple have sensors connected to computer readouts of EEG activity that can establish whether or not a concussion or sub-concussive event has occurred. Although The American Academy of Pain Medicine estimates that nearly 100 million people in the U.S. alone are in chronic pain. Ibuprofen or opioids, even if they can subdue the pain for a while, they don't correct the torsion, compression, fascial or adhesion restrictions, impingements, or disrupted fluid dynamics in the system. Pain medication is very often the treatment of choice for head trauma along with anti-depressants for blast injuries, which can be very complex.

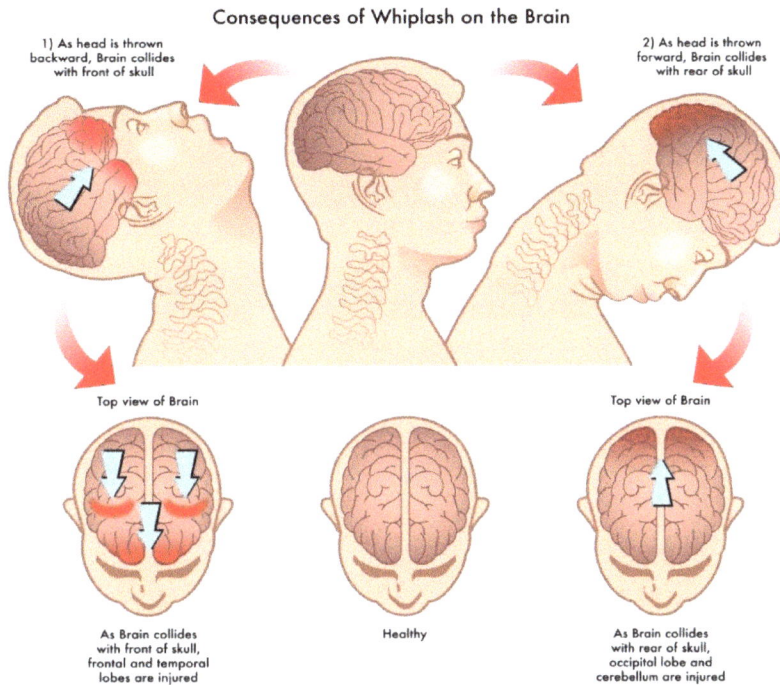

Consequences of Whiplash on the Brain

1) As head is thrown backward, Brain collides with front of skull

2) As head is thrown forward, Brain collides with rear of skull

Top view of Brain

Top view of Brain

As Brain collides with front of skull, frontal and temporal lobes are injured

Healthy

As Brain collides with rear of skull, occipital lobe and cerebellum are injured

Blast injuries create shear and strain forces due to rapidly moving waves that then recede and so suddenly alter the barometric pressure from high to low, so the fluid and air-filled structures are very vulnerable to injury. In addition, there may be other layers of injury from flying objects, toxic chemical substances, and rapid acceleration and deceleration in an explosion, creating coup/contrecoup similar to whiplash injuries. Using pain medication alone cannot remedy all these different dimensions of disorganization. There are ways to limit cell damage and death after a brain injury, as well as to promote the growth of new cells that should be included in each rehab protocol.

Perhaps due to cumulative injuries, perhaps due to size and weight and force differentials or other factors, a Boston University study of the brains of former high school, college, semi-pro, and NFL players had shown progressive indications of CTE starting at a young age. The high school players showed 21% incidence of the disease, semi-pro players exhibited a 64% rate, whereas 91% of college and 99% of NFL players had contracted CTE. At the pre-high school level there was no indication of CTE. However, younger players seem to be more at risk for serious damage and less likely to be seen as in jeopardy. In some instances concussions in young players can even be fatal.

As recently as October, 2018, a 16 year-old football player in Georgia died after a bad hit during a game with uncontrollable swelling and bleeding in the brain. In May of 2018 a young rugby player in Canada died of a brain bleed after colliding with the head of another player, and a 17 year-old female rugby player died a few days after ignoring back-to-back concussions (in the same week) from Second Injury Syndrome. In each case there were periods after the hit when the students felt fine, then collapsed later. Rugby and soccer players don't have helmets so will be less able to have instruments to detect levels of damage.

Deaths close to the concussive event are not as common as a gradual decline in both physical and emotional areas. Researchers discovered that whether there were mild or severe changes in the brain, all exhibited symptoms of "depression, anxiety, memory loss, disinhibition, and other mood or behavior impairments." (Mez, Daneshvar et al, *Clinicopathological Evaluation of Chronic Traumatic Encephalopathy in Players of American Football,* JAMA, July 2017) Young players themselves have been heard saying that they didn't want to know the risks because they wanted to keep playing without worrying about it. Therefore, I think that providing handouts and in-service for parents of athletes, or some form of education should be made available to families in advance so that they're aware of the risks and of what to look for as possible signs of brain injury.

What do the brains of players look like who have sub-clinical hits on a regular basis? SPECT and PET scans show promise in this regard, and have already been used by Dr. Daniel Amen in thousands of cases of head trauma from all causes. Doctors Bazarian, Blyth, and Cimpello wrote an article on their findings of post-concussive syndrome. They defined concussions as forces causing deformation of the brain after coming into contact with the rigid skull after a sudden acceleration or deceleration from an accident, blow, or fall. Bazarian's researchers were making a case for the use of more detailed imaging to find the areas of damage that will not show on a CT scan which mainly looks for a bleed.

 The time frame in these cases being one month after the injury, showed on an MRI as having increased activity in the right parietal and right dorsolateral frontal regions during a complex memory task compared to their controls. The test interpretation along with reports from participants indicated that the injured group had to work harder to pull from working memory. *("Bench to Bedside: Evidence for Brain Injury after Concussion; Looking Beyond the Computed Tomography Scan",* Academic Emergency Medicine, 2006).

I certainly still feel the struggle at times in my brain to take in and process new visual information for taking or teaching a class, for writing books, or for completing paperwork in general. In a different study by Bazarian of concussed patients with normal CT scans, between 59% and 87% presented with abnormal SPECT scans. In these cases the abnormalities were found in the frontal lobes, basal ganglia, temporal lobes, or thalamus weeks or months after the injury, as well as "substantial derangement of cytoskeleton elements of damaged axons". It will it be easier to create appropriate treatment when a more accurate diagnostic is routinely available. There's also a possibility that the scan results would vary according to when it was taken. Symptoms can also shift over time, with many of the cognitive and balance issues showing up later.

As far as some of the neurophysiological changes after a concussion, these researchers reported:

"After a blow to the head, proteins released from the breakdown of neuronal axons and neuronal supporting cells such as astrocytes diffuse into the cerebrospinal fluid, cross the blood-brain barrier, and reach the peripheral circulation where they can be detected. Neuronal proteins studied in the context of concussion include neuron-specific enolase and cleaved tau. Astrocyte and oligodendrocyte proteins studied include S-100B, creatine kinase BB isoenzyme, glial fibrillary acidic protein, and myelin basic protein."

There were other serum markers released in the case of the most severe TBI's that were not present in the more mild to moderate concussions. The S100B marker may be the most often studied due to its presence in Alzheimer's, Down's syndrome, and schizophrenia. However more sensitive testing methods have found the marker to be present in 77% of 122 concussions, and elevated levels were also seen in hockey, basketball, and soccer players, as well as long distance runners. Concussion patients with high levels were twice as likely to report post-concussion symptoms up to a year later. Compromise in balance consistent with axonal damage was shown objectively to be present from 5 to 80 months after the injury.

These results were on test subjects who received no treatment following the injury, so there may indeed be a much better prognosis if some measures were taken right after to help settle the nervous system, balance the brain, optimize motion of the cranial bones once again, and offer brain nutrition. Leg strength, swallowing, balance and mental capacity were increased in my mother two years after she suffered nine cerebral vascular accidents using brain nutrition, oxygen, physical therapy, chiropractic, and acupuncture. Five years later, when she'd stopped speaking and was put on a feeding tube due to fear for her risk of pneumonia from faulty swallowing, she finally said, "I can talk, I'm just weak."

Loss of energy is a huge part of the aging process and likely even more of a concern in those who've had brain injury where neurophysiological and biomechanical alterations have taken place. There has been much more attention paid to regaining cellular energy in recent years. Moreira, Carvalho, et al stated in a 2010 article on the subject that, *"Mitochondria are uniquely poised to play a pivotal role in neuronal cell survival or death because they are regulators of both energy metabolism and cell death pathways."* (*"Mitochondrial dysfunction is a trigger of Alzheimer's disease pathophysiology"*, Science Direct, Vol. 1802, Jan. 2010). Along these lines, Dr. McKee believes that *"improved treatment will come through understanding the physical changes in the brain that occur at the microscopic and molecular levels when the brain is subject to trauma."* A 2017 article published in the Journal of Biological Psychiatry states that, *"Pain experienced over a long period of time can cause rewiring and remodeling of the nervous system, leading to a chronic pain syndrome."*

The causes, as laid out by this article are either that a pain fiber is damaged releasing growth factors and macrophages at the site, whereby new axons become attached to the same dorsal horn leading to "non-painful stimuli being interpreted as pain"; or after prolonged stimulation of C fibers leading to increased release of presynaptic glutamate, activation of post-synaptic AMPA receptors, along with a cascade of additional biochemical and gene transcription alterations that induce prolonged or repetitive pain signals.

Anthony Dickenson in his 2016 article on *"The Neurobiology of Chronic Pain States"*, reports that *"Peripheral nerves can become sensitized, spinal cord neurons can be rendered hyper-excitable, and ascending projections to higher centers can further trigger changes in descending controls from the midbrain and brainstem."* This same plasticity that can modify relationships to stimuli that produce persistent pain states can also be employed to reverse them. Exercise that oxygenates and reeducates the system can be the difference in how much or how long pain is felt.

Females and Injuries

Another fact that can change for the better with more awareness is that female bodies react differently to concussions and head injuries than males do. Their symptoms tend to be more severe and last longer (American Medical Society for Sports Medicine position statement: *"Concussion in Sport"*, 2012), they sustain more head injuries in sports (Dick & Angel 2007; A E Lincoln et. al, 2012), and are more vulnerable to injury. Current thinking is that this fact is possibly due to weaker neck muscles and greater forces generated by angle and acceleration (Medicine and Science Sports and Exercise Journal, 2005), and the influence of hormone levels on cognition and connective tissue. (Journal of Head Trauma Rehabilitation, 2014)

Females are also more likely to report a head injury than their male counterparts. Apparently estrogen is a pain modulator while progesterone supports cognitive function and each plays a role in muscle tone, so it is understandable that from puberty onwards, females begin to sustain more injuries and experience more pain. The Harvard Health Blog (Schmerling, 2015) suggests that another contributing factor for increased injuries in females is that a wider pelvis changes the alignment through the knee (knee injuries 2-6X more frequent in females), and that they land differently after jumping. Estrogen also plays a role in muscle tension, muscle energy, and muscle cell energy metabolism. A study by the University of Jyväskyiä in Finland (October, 2017) showed that the drop in the female steroid hormone estradiol during menopause makes female athletes much more vulnerable to stress fractures around middle age as hormone levels begin to change, and as muscle size and strength are likely to decrease. Lower levels of estrogen generate higher levels of cortisol which can raise blood pressure and blood sugar and also generate increased muscle tension with consequential fatigue and anxiety. Progesterone, the hormone that would attenuate the tension from reduced estrogen levels, also begins to drop creating the common complaint from seniors of those stiff joints and general aches and pains. On the contrary, younger female athletes are at risk during their cycle when hormonal levels are high and ligaments become lax, and joints become unstable. While some female athletes are choosing to use birth control pills to help stabilize the hormone levels, there may be other concerns raised here.

Structural differences also account for additional vulnerability in women. Females also have less muscle mass, they have more fat, decreased bone density, and greater flexibility in general which makes quick changes in direction more hazardous. For those approaching or cruising through menopause, the drop in estrogen stimulates leaky guy which produces inflammation which also leads to increased breakdown in bone. In this regard, workouts for women would need to be geared more toward strengthening the areas that would make them more prone to injury, and perhaps consider taping areas that could benefit from additional support. Much of what needs to be emphasized here is that during an impact injury, many layers of the system become dysregulated, some of which are cells that are responsible for regulating other functions. The issues may show up in endocrine or fluid systems whereby there's an alteration in blood pressure, in lymph flow, or even in menses.

There's usually some significant pain, which can distract the sufferer from noticing the other imbalances, and give the impression that once the pain subsides that all is well. That's why it's so helpful to visit a practitioner who's familiar with tracking and treating the many layers or regions of imbalance. Evidence shows that hormonal systems can both become dysregulated as well as become the source of imbalance. Therefore, seeing someone in osteopathy or having a more global assessment through a functional medicine doctor could prevent systemic issues from cropping up later on. Manual medicine practitioners can also make adjustments to visceral and fluid bodies. It should not be assumed that by receiving treatment for the brain alone that the other systems will automatically self-correct, nor that treating the peripheral areas will automatically correct the brain.

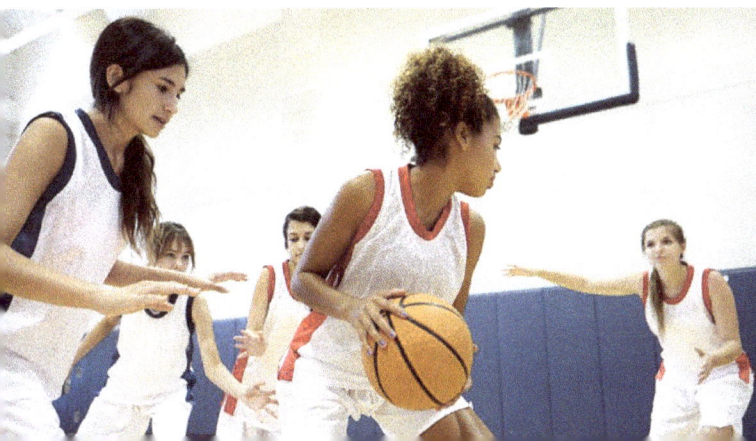

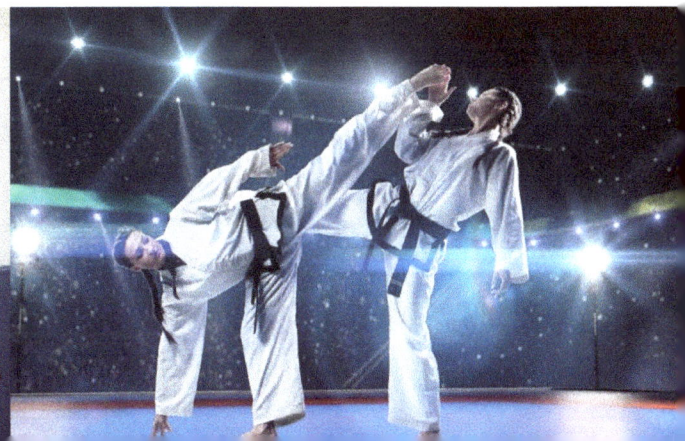

Each system should be assessed and treated individually in relationship to the functioning of the whole. The symptoms can easily overlap with other aspects of life that could seem like the cause. For example irritability or mood changes can be seen as disappointment with a losing streak or stressful job rather than being attributed to an injury to the head. I heard of another case where a family may knew that their uncle was a happy-go-lucky person until a fall off a horse put him in a bad mood ever since, but no one knew that anything could be done about it. His main residual was a mood disorder. We now know that EMDR, low-frequency neurofeedback, diet, and microbiome modifications can all have a positive effect on mood disorders. Everyone won't experience personality changes, but it's still a good idea to seek proper assessment using a multi-disciplinary approach since a variety of systems can be impacted by an accident, fall, or injury. It could have affected immune efficiency, vascular sufficiency, detox capabilities, cognitive functioning, or stress levels, but was misappropriated to unknown or other causes and accepted as the new norm.

It would be like trying to reach a destination when there are so many detours you wind up in a different place without a road map. In my case there were so many instances of nausea after a head injury that went away after working with my neck, I understood not to look for it in the belly. The body couldn't give me the proper source of the nausea, but luckily I knew where to look from experience not to look for an allergy or some other culprit. Some leftover from the injuries produced vulnerability for inflammation near C 3-4, and it could be that the vagus nerve got irritated in the process and upset the belly. Nausea is a common symptom in head injuries, but not one you'd expect to last years later.

I'm hoping that sharing some of these details in how the after-effects of concussions can present themselves long after the initial event, that many types of post-concussive symptoms can be demystified. When neither you nor your practitioner are familiar enough with the mild to moderate dysfunctions that can cause all types of annoying discomforts, you'll more likely repress them and get on with your day. Remember that an already compromised system will be more vulnerable to reactivity of any origin, be it viral, emotional, allergens, or new injuries, since your healing powers have been diminished, communication between systems compromised, and it takes more effort and energy for your brain to perform simple tasks. It may not be that you're getting older, it may be that your brain hasn't fully healed yet.

Traumatic Brain Injury Symptoms

Brains of those who've suffered concussions frequently show damage in the frontal and temporal lobes because those areas are where the brain is closer to the rigid bone it hits, according to Dr. James Kelly, professor of neurosurgery. In addition, Dr. Thomas McCann finds that: *"Linear translation and rotational forces, which in combination produce angular acceleration or deceleration, can result in the straining, shearing, and compression of brain*

Superior sagittal sinus

Skin of scalp

Periosteum

Hair

Bone of skull

Periosteal layer

Meningeal layer

Dura mater

Arachnoid mater

Pia mater

Subdural space

Subarachnoid space

Gray matter

White matter

Brain

Falx cerebri

Blood vessel

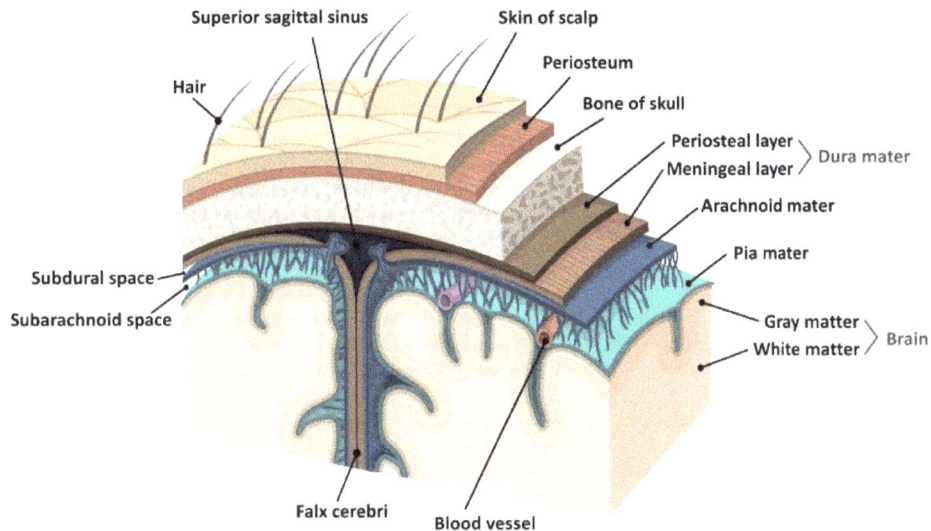

tissue in a TBI." Secondary symptoms often show up days or months after the initial injury, making it more difficult for families to attribute the issues to the original injury.

McCann finds that the brain areas most vulnerable to these forces are the cerebellum, the ventral brain stem (where RAS lives), the entorhinal/hippocampal complex, the amygdala, temporal polar cortex, orbitofrontal cortex (involved in emotional and social responses), and dorsolateral prefrontal cortex where problem solving and so many of our other executive functions take place. (Dialogues in Clinical Neuroscience, "*Neurobiological consequences of traumatic brain injury*", 2011)

Stecco describes a fascial mechanism whereby the chronic, hypersensitivity with injuries can manifest and may be the most challenging aspect. He reports, "*Under normal physiological conditions, the elasticity of the fascia allows it to adapt to compression without straining the free nerve endings. Normally the free nerve endings are involved in deep somaesthetic activity or the perception of the body's position and movement in space. In pathological conditions, such as in the presence of a densification of the fascia, these free nerve endings are under tension which tends to lower their pain threshold. In such a situation even a minimal compression can be sufficient to override the threshold, setting off local pain as well as referred pain.*" (Luigi Stecco, Fascial Manipulation for Musculoskeletal Pain, 2004) Most manual therapists can remember cases when even a light touch produces tenderness.

I'd experienced so many back-to-back head injuries at one point that I could almost predict which symptoms were yet to come. The sensitization to pain was probably one of the worst trigger-happy outcomes, and the areas along the path of the transverse cervical nerve were the most tenacious. They say that 75% of the healing takes place in the first year, and 25% of what is left that is amenable to healing will happen in the second year. Whether or not these results can change based upon immediacy of intervention remains to be seen and would be a worthwhile investigation to make. In my case, as I became more familiar with the symptoms and how to address them, the time for resolution became shorter, and in fact additional healing continues to happen years later.

The catch-22 is that sleep is probably the best healer for the cognitive issues and it's very difficult to sleep deeply when the brain is dysregulated. I've never taken sleeping pills and didn't like the feeling the next day when I tried melatonin or valerian. I did, through the grapevine, hear that tart cherry juice increases the body's production of melatonin and taking some before bed did help. Chamomile tea, various sleeping teas, hot baths, and magnesium also helped a lot. I'd heard very recently that nutmeg had sedative qualities, so adding that to a calming tea before bed actually did produce a deeper sleep.

Pathologist, Dr. Omalu, who was one of the first to publicize his concern over Chronic Traumatic Encephaly, received calls from concerned parents in the wake of his findings when they began noticing behavioral changes in their teenagers. (Rachel Alexander, <u>Athletic Business</u>, 2018) As alarming as it was to discover the intensity of the damage and changes in a person's temperament, mental stability, cognitive capacity, and personality in these older pro ball players, when an 18 year-old young athlete's brain was examined, they discovered he had the brain of a person decades older. The Mayo clinic found in a study conducted in 2015 that a certain percentage of those showing early signs of the condition hadn't played sports, but experienced a *single fall or accident* years earlier.

Mild Brain Injury Symptoms (According to the Mayo Clinic

- fatigue
- headaches
- visual disturbances
- poor attention/concentration
- memory loss
- sleep disturbances
- dizziness and loss of balance
- irritability
- emotional disturbances
- feelings of depression
- seizures
- nausea
- loss of smell
- sensitivity to light and sound
- mood changes/swings
- getting lost or confused
- slowed thinking

Symptoms of moderate to severe TBI can include:
- persistent or worsening headaches
- repeated vomiting or nausea
- convulsions or seizures
- dilated pupils
- fluids draining from nose or ears
- sleep disturbances
- loss of coordination
- weakness or numbness in fingers and toes
- slurred speech
- agitation
- combativeness, aggression
- loss of consciousness

With increasing intensity that correlates to the number of incidents, I can say with certainty that I've experienced at least 90% of these symptoms from the mild through the severe categories. They must have persisted longer because during some periods there were several mild ones on top of more serious injuries in a single year. Although it's very important for one injury to have time to heal before a new trauma occurs, it wasn't the case in my circumstance. Partially due to the fact that reduced spatial orientation and awareness along with balance issues follow head trauma, and partially due to the small and low ceilings and beams I needed to navigate in the work space without good bearings, it just kept happening.

In addition to those listed above, I also experienced ADHD, PTSD, brain fatigue, significant throat tension with the prolonged use of the eyes, thoracic outlet syndrome, vaso-vagal reactions, dyslexia, REM sleep disorder, difficulty lifting my arms and legs, and expressive aphasia, whereby what comes out of your mouth doesn't match what you were perceiving and intending to say. The example that made me aware I'd better seek treatment was the time I looked up at the sky at a bird and remarked, "I didn't know turkeys could swim!" Right after laughing at myself I began to research head trauma remedies. The pain had been long gone, but the cognitive issues had begun to surface and multiply. I also had debilitating dyslexia whereby phone numbers, addresses, dates and times were reversed or completely confused.

I'd missed flights because I just couldn't figure out the time of departure even though staring at the numbers on the ticket and thinking I'd calculated the time to get to the airport was right. At times I confused the arrival time with the departure time while being relieved that I'd gotten to the airport on time. A little shock hit my system when I realized that the flight had already left. It'd be funny if it weren't so darn inconvenient for you and the person waiting to pick you up. One airline agreed to not penalize me for the no-show (when I showed up the wrong day) if I brought a doctor's note. After so many of these experiences, some anxiety began to form about going anywhere.

So it's not just an inaccessible type of confusion that sets in that makes the post-concussion stage difficult, it's that you don't realize you're confused until it's pointed out by something or someone outside of yourself. You can't catch it in time. You not only notice yourself losing track of your daily flow of life, but you notice losing track of yourself. I began forgetting and losing so many things and losing time, or forgetting that I'd remembered something and act like I'd forgotten it all over again, I got anxious every time I was about to leave the house or travel. Eventually I was able to be more relaxed about forgetting, and at some point devised strategies to help remember the most important things.

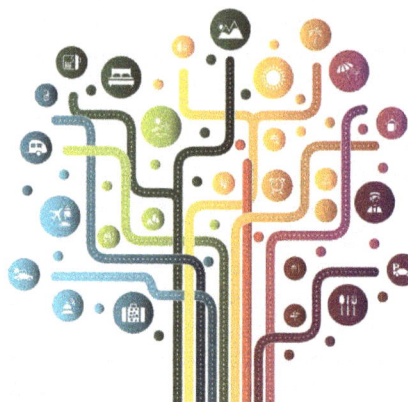

There was also a sense of blacking out while awake that is hard to explain, but it's like a mini-seizure or an episode where you're just not on board with your brain and its ability to process through the senses and logical mind. When you come back to, there's a sense of, "What just happened? Was I in the middle of something?" It sounds like the jokes seniors tell about not remembering why came into a room, but who in their 50's wants the brain of someone 20 years older? To overcome this symptom I began talking to myself on the way to do something in another room so it would stay in my mind long enough to stay on purpose, and that worked well. Somehow engaging the faculty of hearing was a great support to the memory process, and slowly, slowly muscle memory began to return.

The brain and non-ionizing radiation

The environmental triggers in modern society can make the sensitive rehabilitation process even more challenging, as they further dysregulate the brain. Non-ionizing radiation, of the type that is emitted by smart meters, microwaves, and cell phones have been shown to penetrate the brains of young children far more than those in their teen or adult years. Pregnant women are 30-40% more at risk for cell death in the fetus and loss of the pregnancy. But researchers now know that there are fluctuation/pulsing issues with the emanations that are different than just heating issues and happen at a rate that is 600x above EPA acceptable levels. (Dr. Dietrich Klinghardt, 2016) Similar to brain injury, radiation from very high to extremely low frequencies "can interfere with the biological processes of cell communication and cell metabolism" along with creating oxidative stress and increased permeability of the blood brain barrier that have been shown to cause disease. (Mensch, et al, Internationaler Ärteappell, 2012) The U.S. Navy conducted over 2300 studies as far back as the 1970's on the dangers of non-ionizing radiation by microwaves and radio frequencies which they discovered evidence of the following:

- Heating of the organs: including the whole body, skin, bone and bone marrow, lens of the eye and cornea, genitalia, brain, sinuses, and metal implants
- Changes in physiologic function including: contraction of striated muscles, dilation of blood vessels, changes to oxidative processes in tissues and organs, liver impairment, decreased fertility, altered menstrual activity, altered fetal development, altered renal function, decreased electrical resistance on the skin, and altered blood flow

More recent studies on the effects of wifi at 2.45 Ghz names (current phones are at 4 Ghz) these frequencies as major risk factors for brain tumors and other neurodegenerative conditions (Dasdag, et al, International Journal of Radiation Biology, 2015), in addition to having negative effects on the brain's glucose metabolism. (Volkow, et al, JAMA, 2012) Some of the symptoms with just short term exposure are reported as being: headaches, irregular or racing heartbeat, nausea, fatigue, tinnitus, insomnia, inflammation, memory problems, high blood pressure, muscle twitching, difficulty concentrating, impaired immunity, and more, adding to the challenges to heal from head trauma, as many of the stressors and resulting symptoms are the same. Brain patients are likely more vulnerable to this radiation, as are many who have or have had chronic health issues.

Reducing whatever other stressors that may impact health will be in service of the brain's healing process. There are doctors who feel that the brain won't heal without correcting the balance in the belly. A new field of neuropsychiatry has sprung up that focuses on brain nutrition and mental states. A change in diet can serve the brain directly and indirectly by supporting better mood, by feeding the brain, and by supporting the heart. There's an entire field of study now called neurocardiolgy after the discovery that the heart has most of the neurotransmitters that the brain has (and so does the gut). Some professionals feel that anything that helps the heart will also help the brain. Although many systems can become dysregulated with a brain injury, there are also many doors through which it can be helped by supporting related systems.

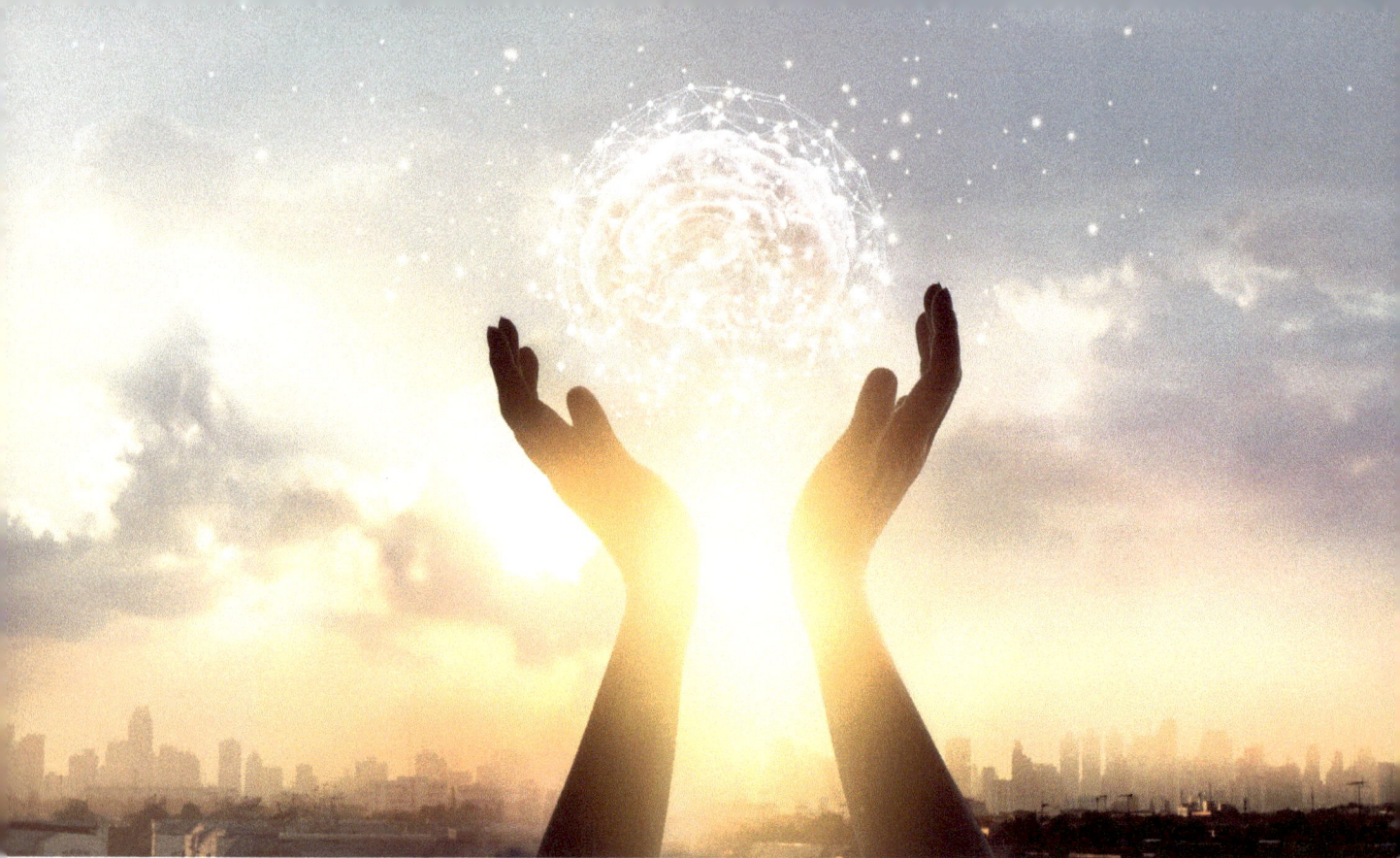

Chapter 3

The Brain is a Miracle Ready to Happen

"The conventional approach is really very deficient and will often leave people with cognitive deficits or, what we call a decline in brain reserve. We all have a certain amount of brain reserve whether it's a kid or adult, but if there's brain injury and it's not taken care of appropriately, then the person's brain reserve can go down. If it goes down enough, they'll start having symptoms."

~ Dr. Norman Doidge (Broken Brain, Ep.6)

Just a little about this amazing bundle of intelligence

The brain is composed of nearly 75% water and 60% fat with blood vessels that could reach over 100,000 miles if stretched end to end. It uses about 20% of the body's blood and 20% of its oxygen at any given moment during a normal day, and around the same percentage of the body's energy. It is comprised of grey matter which contains between 80-90 billion neurons, with about 100 trillion glial or perineural cells, according to von Barheld, Bahney, & Houzel, preciously thought to be a fraction of that ratio. (Journal of Comparative Neurology, May, 2016)

The white matter contains trillions of axons and dendrites that are myelinated and therefore generate millisecond transmissions to other parts of the brain. They are the vital connections that facilitate optimal brain function and are found to be responsible for neurodegenerative conditions when damaged, either through the protective sheath being compromised, tau protein buildup, or through the tearing and over-stretching that happens in traumatic brain injury. Recent studies have recently shown that structural changes in the white matter after learning a new skill, including the volume, anatomical organization, and functional connectivity tracts linking to cortical areas for visual-motor control or reading being increased, depending upon the activity the subjects focused on (R. Douglas Fields, *Science Magazine*, Nov. 2016). It was previously thought that only grey matter, not white matter exhibited neuroplasticity, yet the oligodendrites thereon were shown to have an influence in consolidating memory while asleep during developmental stages of the brain.

The fatty myelin sheath that surrounds these nerve fibers conducts electrical impulses, and when the wiring becomes faulty, or scarred/sclerotic as in multiple sclerosis, the resulting inflammation can cause intense pain, contractions anywhere in the body, dropped foot syndrome, blindness, and more, should the disease progress. Dr. Chris Iliades writes about a study (Annals of Neurology, Calabrese et al July, 2013) that was able to predict with 88% accuracy which 400 patients would progress in their MS diagnosis by observing brain volume alone, even though brain shrinkage is 'normal' with age. At the height of my concern for my future following a serious concussion in 2000, I had an MRI at Kaiser which showed hyper-intensity of the white matter "consistent with MS". I believed it was from the head injury and not deterioration of the sheath due to inflammation or scarring, although I couldn't prove it and kept my fingers crossed.

I declined to start medication and felt both inspired and a little worried I'd heard later than another woman who'd had migraines had an MRI with this hyper-intensity. Was the axonal tearing creating the migraines? Were the migraines creating the hyper-intensity? It was still a puzzle. The doctor told me to come back if the symptoms got worse. I didn't go back. I rejected the diagnosis and became more determined to find a solution.

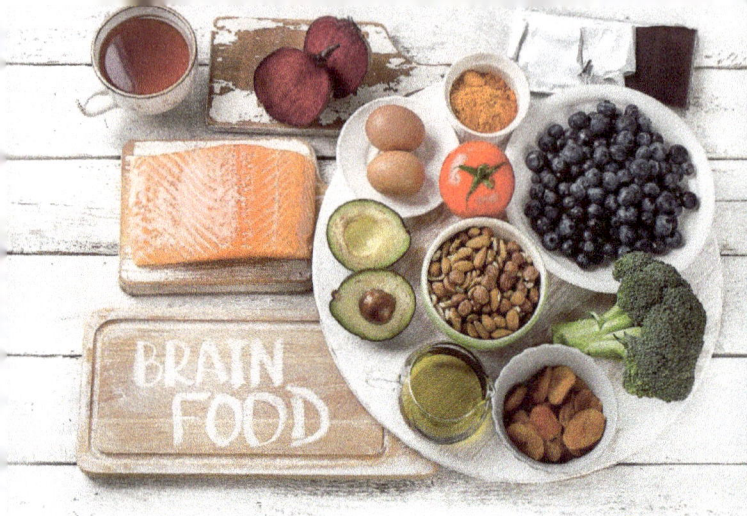

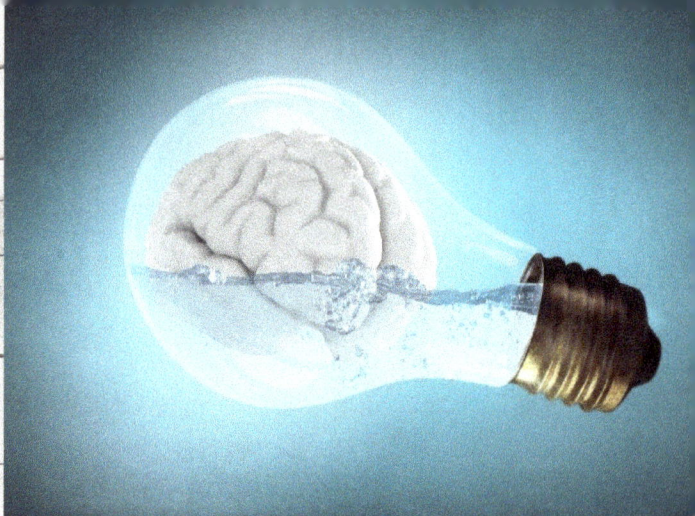

The brain needs nutrition to function optimally, even if it hasn't been injured. I can only imagine that the injured brain requires even more of a nutritional focus when it's trying to heal. A study led by Dr. Dale Bredesen was able to reverse symptoms of mild cognitive decline or early Alzheimer's in 10 volunteers using diet, exercise, sleep, brain stimulation, and various vitamins and supplements. My symptoms also dissipated using those same ingredients, although not his protocol specifically. Though not true for everyone, my system desperately needed red meat to get stronger. A decent night's sleep took a while to cultivate, but the rest was invaluable. Meditation helped make up for the lack of sleep.

It's good to realize that as far as brain shrinkage goes, mild dehydration can not only significantly reduce the brain volume, but can produce serious symptoms that could get easily misunderstood or missed. Since nerve conduction is electrical and water is a significant medium of conductivity, and that its conductivity requires half of the brain's energy, dehydration can have dire consequences. Some of the symptoms can include reduced focus and memory, brain fatigue and brain fog, headaches, sleep issues, anger, and depression. Sound familiar? A study on brain hydration performed by the Georgia Institute of Technology, showed "complex problem-solving, coordination, and attention suffered the most." Apparently, one reason that elders are more vulnerable to dehydration is because they don't sense thirst as easily. This is a brain deficit cause with a simple solution: set up a schedule.

The Brain and Consciousness

"I hold that he brain is the most powerful organ of the human body... wherefore I assert that the brain is the interpreter of consciousness" – Hippocrates

Most of the activity of the brain is unconscious, yet whether we are aware of its functions or not, it's been confirmed that hydration, nutrition, exercise, and sleep support it being able to perform well at all. Under normal conditions, what the brain can achieve is nothing less than miraculous. Some estimates go as high as hundreds of trillions of calculations and perceptions that happen every second in the brain without our knowledge, whereas the conscious mind can only be aware of a handful of processes each second. There are even books written on how to let your less-than-conscious perceptions run the show since they can process large quantities of information even before it reaches the conscious mind. We have organ systems that perceive and interpret info before it reaches the brain. But what is it that makes anyone conscious of the information the gut, heart, or mind can receive?

Professor Dr. Gerhard Ruhenstorth-Bauer at the Max-Plank Institute describes consciousness as, "*Consciousness is the state or quality of awareness, or of being aware of an external object or something within oneself.*" It has been defined as "sentience, awareness, subjectivity, the ability to experience or feel, wakefulness, having a sense of selfhood, and the executive control system of the mind." I would posit that using the ability to be self-aware or in the best way, self-conscious, has a profound effect on health, well-being, and the injury recovery process. We may never nail down a specific explanation of how our many types of intelligence are able to function, but it's helpful to access as much of it as you can.

The many different interpretations of what constitutes consciousness depend upon which field of study is doing the interpreting. Perhaps many of the conflicting descriptions would dissipate into complementary ones if consciousness was seen as being limitless, fluid, and multi-dimensional in how it is able to manifest. Spiritual paths can also define consciousness differently and point to a state that is beyond the waking, sleeping, or dreaming states of consciousness.

Larry Dossey, M.D. has written a few books on the subject of 'non-local mind' and states that, "*The concept that consciousness is a fundamental, unitary, collective entity is ancient. It is traceable to wisdom traditions that are at least 3,000 years old. My interest in this idea, however, arose from empirical evidence that has been accumulating for more than a century. In brief, this evidence suggests that a linkage exists between individual minds that transcends separation in both space and time. This evidence profoundly suggests that individual minds can communicate and exchange information at arbitrary distances, into the future or the past.*"

Who or what is driving consciousness in the first place? Is the brain the master or the servant, or is something else organizing how it functions? What parts do belief and intention play in what shows up in structures or their functions? Biologist Bruce Lipton, author of "Biology of Belief", would say that belief plays a huge role in how a system will respond to any situation because he's shown that our cells react to beliefs. Placebos are also a splendid example of this phenomena. Does karma play a part? Spiritual teacher and Yogi Master Vasudev states, "*Unless you take control of your destiny, your life will be in the hands of fate.*" Then there's Carl Jung's similar quote, "*Unless you make the unconscious conscious, it will direct your life and you will call it fate.*"

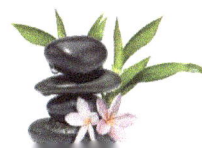

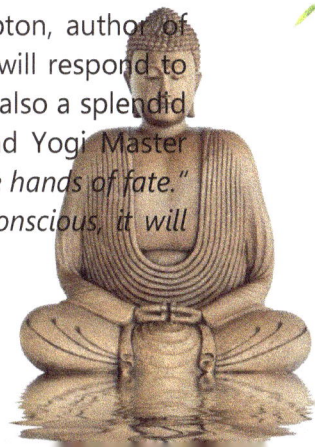

In a 2015 article entitled, "What is Consciousness? A Mystic's Perspective", Satguru Vasudev explains it this way:

"We call this intelligence that makes life happen consciousness. The only reason you experience aliveness is because you are conscious…. What we refer to as consciousness is a much subtler dimension of who you are, and it is commonly shared by everyone. It is the same intelligence that is turning food into flesh in me, in you, in everyone. If we move people being identified with the boundaries of their physical body to a deeper dimension within themselves, their sense of 'me' and 'you' decreases; 'you' and 'I' are seen to be the same. This means that consciousness has risen on a social level. Essentially, we do not raise consciousness. We raise your experience so that you become more conscious."

Since a view of consciousness can depend upon what someone is able to perceive within its vastness, descriptions will vary. Consciousness is a malleable potential that is both pre-programmed and programmable, both transmitting what it receives, but also capable of altering its transmissions. It can also be seen as the field from which anything arises. The brain, as well as consciousness, has an enormous potential for multi-dimensional or multi-modal expression. It can appear as limitless creativity, as extra-sensory capacities like Larry Dossey expressed, and as abilities beyond the body's normal functions like yogis and martial arts and spiritual Masters have achieved. For example, well-known sage Poonjaji normalized his own blood sugar many times when anyone else would have been in a diabetic coma. Swami Nisargadatta was reported to have shown that he was unaffected by LSD, as anyone in normal consciousness would have been.

Some cultures use concepts like the 99 names of Nothingness to describe the many faces of God, or the variety of ways that consciousness can express itself. Within certain cultures there may be a deity named for a particular quality like compassion, or abundance, fertility, war, creativity, healing, and so on. It seems that spiritual seekers and finders from various cultures were finding ways to reveal that there are endless possibilities for how this ever-present intelligence can express itself. If we focus on being more aware of this intelligence residing in us, we can find that space in us beneath where the symptoms are generate Many ancient as well as more current traditions can bring the body out of the trance-like, auto-pilot state of functioning into which it has become conditioned. This is different than the brain fog that comes with head trauma. Brain fog from injury can be helped by a broader awakening in the potentialities of consciousness. Using methods like meditation or Chi Kung to increase energy or enhance the self-sensing abilities of the system can begin to reveal many of the other layers of perception.

A large part of Feldenkrais or Hanna Somatics, Elsa Gindler's Sensory Awareness practices, and also Matthias Alexander's remarkable reports of healing come from techniques that wake up self-awareness to that inner intelligence, presenting in one way as that greater capacity for what consciousness can do. Ancient systems like Chinese Medicine and Chi kung find that imbalances show up in the energetic systems a while before they create symptoms in physical structures or physiological functions.

In this vein it's conceivable that contemplative practices or energetic balancing will influence the trajectory of injuries on many levels and could make a difference in recovery. In my case the lines between some aspects of the subconscious, unconscious, and conscious mind and body were becoming blurred. It actually seemed like the part of me that was being driven to become more conscious was the 'unconscious' part. It also felt like the unconscious part was connected to a whole universe of possibilities beyond logic that the conscious mind could eventually appreciate and begin to sense more and more.

I had a feeling that the answers to chronic conditions might lay in the mystery that doesn't get taught in the school systems, but that Dr. Wonderly was pointing to without elucidating. I had a feeling that the consequences of my past accidents and choices could be overcome by what that awakening intelligence could communicate to my being. I may not have an accurate or a scientific explanation for exactly how that intelligence is able to communicate, but at some point I could feel that the movement of consciousness was opening and releasing energy, shifting fascia, and balancing joint positions. It also shifted muscular tensions, lifted my mood and cleared brain fog. This was the beginning of a contemplative and feeling journey alongside of the intellectual one that engaged a different part of the 'brain' and another layer of consciousness.

What Makes the Brain Conscious?

Anatomically, the area of the brain that determines whether you are able to be awake or in a coma has been shown recently by a group of Harvard researchers to lie in the rostral dorsolateral pontine tegmentum. (American Academy of Neurology, Fischer, Boes, Demertzi, et. al, 2016) This small area of the brainstem connects to the ventral anterior insula and pregenual anterior cingulate cortex, and if those connections are disrupted, the ability of a person to regain 'consciousness' is also disrupted. The reticular activating system (RAS) in the mesopons area of the brain stem controls the sleep, three dreaming stages, and waking states.

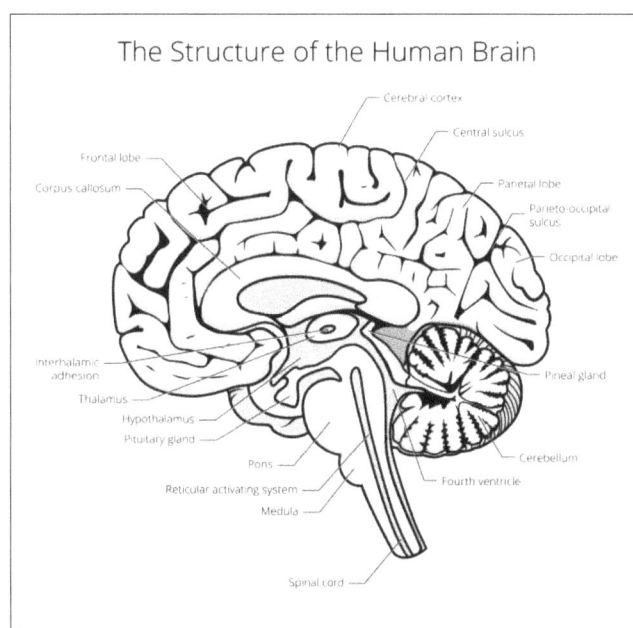

The Structure of the Human Brain

Cerebral cortex
Central sulcus
Frontal lobe
Corpus callosum
Parietal lobe
Parieto-occipital sulcus
Occipital lobe
Interthalamic adhesion
Pineal gland
Thalamus
Hypothalamus
Pituitary gland
Cerebellum
Pons
Fourth ventricle
Reticular activating system
Medula
Spinal cord

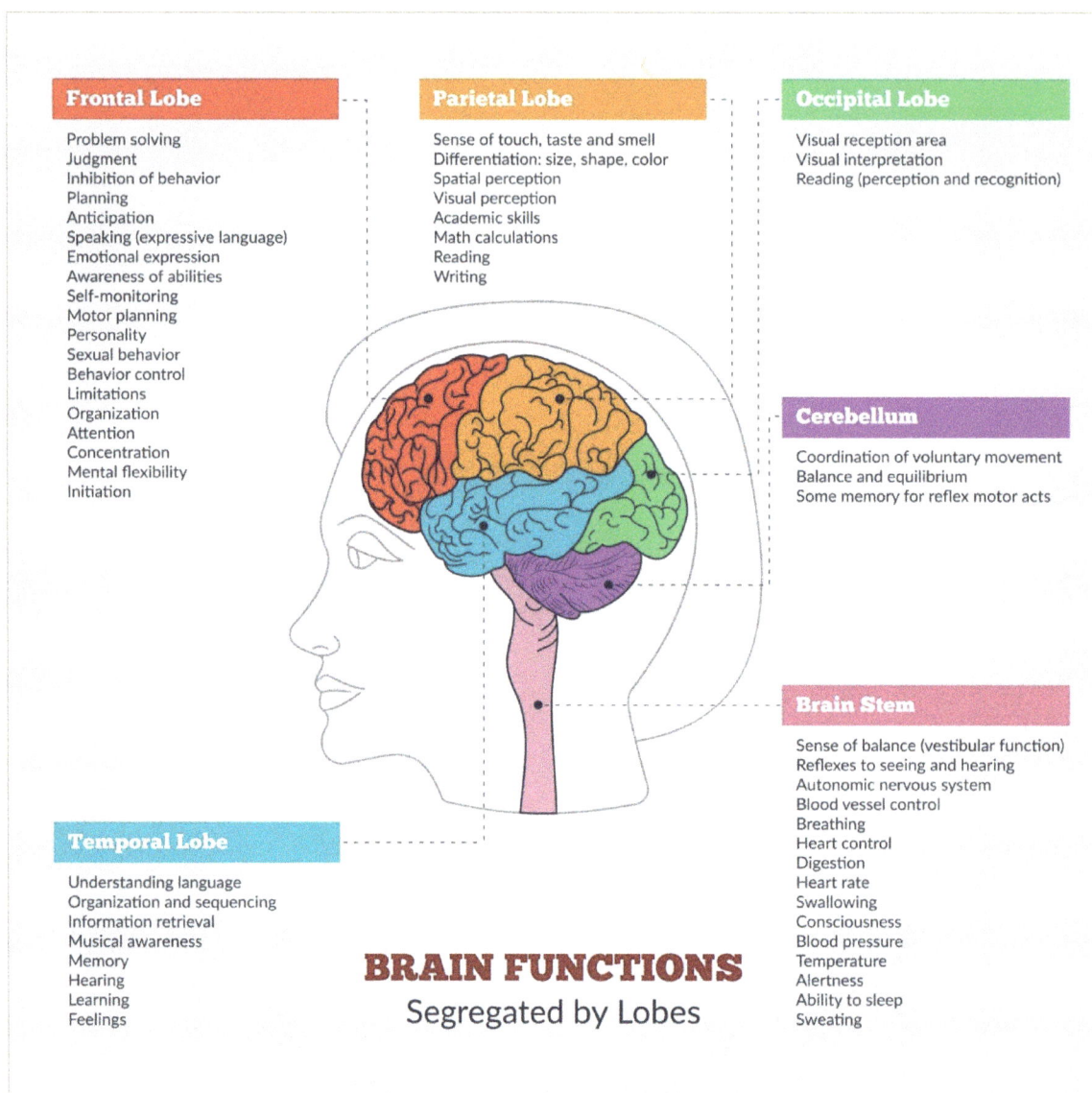

Frontal Lobe

Problem solving
Judgment
Inhibition of behavior
Planning
Anticipation
Speaking (expressive language)
Emotional expression
Awareness of abilities
Self-monitoring
Motor planning
Personality
Sexual behavior
Behavior control
Limitations
Organization
Attention
Concentration
Mental flexibility
Initiation

Parietal Lobe

Sense of touch, taste and smell
Differentiation: size, shape, color
Spatial perception
Visual perception
Academic skills
Math calculations
Reading
Writing

Occipital Lobe

Visual reception area
Visual interpretation
Reading (perception and recognition)

Cerebellum

Coordination of voluntary movement
Balance and equilibrium
Some memory for reflex motor acts

Brain Stem

Sense of balance (vestibular function)
Reflexes to seeing and hearing
Autonomic nervous system
Blood vessel control
Breathing
Heart control
Digestion
Heart rate
Swallowing
Consciousness
Blood pressure
Temperature
Alertness
Ability to sleep
Sweating

Temporal Lobe

Understanding language
Organization and sequencing
Information retrieval
Musical awareness
Memory
Hearing
Learning
Feelings

BRAIN FUNCTIONS
Segregated by Lobes

The RAS links with the descending reticulospinal tracts, with the ascending hypothalamic, the basal forebrain, and thalamocortical systems. (E. Garcia Rill, Encyclopedia of Neuroscience, 2009). In their study the reticular formation was seen to have high connectivity to the lateral prefontal cortex and ventromedial prefrontal cortex, and low connectivity to the primary motor cortex, the premotor cortex, the primary somatosensory motor cortex, orbitofrontal, and posterior parietal cortex (Jang & Kwon, 2015) in healthy subjects. It therefore seems that at the most basic levels of awareness the brain has some direct connections to its sensing and movement powers, along with routings for thought processing.

The premise for consciousness in this anatomical perspective is that a certain amount of arousal is needed for the brain to be able to come to attention and focus for meaningful engagement or learning to be able to happen. Arousal of the RAS is therefore key and fundamental for the brain to be able to be 'awake' enough for it to attend to whatever is in front of it. Dr. Sarah Schoen discovered that children with under- or over-active arousal can benefit from overall stimulation of the RAS system in order to help balance sensory integration disorders (Journal of Occupational Therapy Schools and Early Intervention, 2015). One of the main objectives in helping kids with issues learning in school is to find ways to enable them to pay attention. The medical remedy has been Ritalin, which doesn't resolve the brain dysregulation.

Would they be hyperactive if those early childhood falls had been assessed for possible brain disruptions? While the thalamus is often seen as the main bridge between the unconscious or involuntary autonomic systems and the conscious, more voluntary regions of the brain, it is also often considered to be the bridge between the body and the mind. The RAS transmits several projections to both sensory and motor pathways, including the cerebellum which is a central organizer of motor programs and their execution. The cerebellum also connects to areas of the thalamus up to the cortex, as well as to the midbrain related to survival instincts. From there arousal can provoke relevant emotional responses, and appropriate motor reactions to sensory stimuli, such as vision, pain, touch, and temperature. It's also designed to filter out insignificant vs. priority information that needs to be acted on. If this filtering function is compromised, the decision-making process would be compromised as the flood of input would have no editor.

The cerebellum is a common region for head trauma to land, but may not always be the treatment solution. Just to get an idea of how prevalent head injuries are, estimates are that every day 153 people die from traumatic brain injury. Almost three million each year hit the emergency room, with approximately 5 million living with a disability related to head trauma. Note that these are those who went to the emergency room to seek care, but surely hundreds of thousands more aren't treated or aren't reported, particularly those that happen in the course of playing a sport. Four out of five hospital visits for TBI's were from falls in adults, and almost half were for those 14 years of age and younger. The next leading cause of TBI's is auto accidents. Like myself, probably many residual symptoms in millions of people are ignored or attributed to other causes until the lightbulb goes off. In my case the light bulb was another concussion.

If patients become educated that the brain is almost always impacted in falls, sports, and car crashes, general practitioners and orthopedic specialists will also begin to refer to the appropriate professionals for diagnosis and treatment. The hope here is that more people will report their head injury and seek treatment as awareness increases. Understanding is growing that commonly used screening protocols at hospitals are insufficient to catch where the brain damage may lie, and patients can seek out more detailed scans on their own if their doctors aren't aware. As several researchers have shown, multiple brain nuclei are often compromised during a head injury which have far-reaching, long term effects. It should also be useful to know what the symptoms are, so the tendency to wait it out at any age will be replaced by immediate action as a preventative measure.

As important of an area as the RAS is in orchestrating everyday actions according to interpretation of events, it would seem that down-regulating the stress response after a trauma would also be a primary consideration. Discharging cellular trauma and its cascades of biochemical reactions seems like the first on what could then be a shorter list of engaging the system's resources in the direction of repair and restoration. Communicating safety and using methods that let the body know the threat has been contained or removed makes a big difference in systems opening, softening, and allowing the relaxation response to kick in. Breath can send that message, and for some compression communicates safety; gentle, slow skillful touch, working with the vagus nerve, with viscera, and working in fluid systems all can accomplish this shift.

I'm not sure which brain region is responsible for mechanoreceptors being off line, creating the inability to access an area of soft tissue, as in the sensory-motor amnesia that Dr. Hanna describes. It's also still a mystery to me exactly how the brain can go blank or have kinesthetic blind spots, but seeing as both the basal ganglia and cerebellum are implicated in brain injury, a hyper-, hypo- or numb out situation could likely kick in anywhere. I'm not sure if the soft tissue's proprioception has crashed, or that the area of the brain that would be receiving sensory input from that area is off line, so the phone is ringing, but no one's answering. This was my startling experience in bowling; that I could see my body moving, but couldn't feel it from within. That got better through repeating specific conscious movements during floor exercises, which can also be a super indicator of what's gone offline.

Then I got hit on the top of my head with a basketball - right on the sensory-motor cortex as well as the premotor, primary motor cortex and anterior parietal cortex. It morphed into not being able to sense my right side, but my left was back online. My left side felt dull, my neck and sub-occipital area around the brain stem was badly compressed, but ice and serrapeptase eliminated the suture pain in a couple of days. My game went downhill fast. It went from some of the highest scores ever to some of the lowest. My awareness and attention were up and running, but the mechanics of the brain being able to receive sensory input from that side of the body had been suspended in terms of interoception (sensing itself); exteroception (sensing itself in relation to objects) was fine. The most loss of sensation was throughout the right arm.

I decided to sense into the brain to help remedy the issue rather than using movements that might be sending feedback to a faulty receiver. I sent awareness to the cerebellum, the basal ganglia, the pulvinar at the posterior of the thalamus, the claustrum, and the sensory cortex. Somewhere in between the pulvinar and the sensory cortex a light turned on and my right arm came back online. I could once again feel it in 3-D. My bowling scores went back up and there was much better control of where the ball went. Spatial dyslexia continued to linger since childhood, making it difficult to know right from left. I could see it, but not sense it. I also noticed that many times visual blind spots created an inability to perceive things accurately depending upon where they were in space. Sometimes I'd need to turn my head to catch sight of something that was right in front of me if it was small. Now I'm going to sense into the lingual gyrus and see what that does for the visual field. (Coming back to this exploration, my dreams only woke me up if they became lucid after sensing this gyrus, but blind spots remained.)

The belly brain

In recent years there's been a lot of discussion with research findings about how anxiety and depression can be mitigated by the microbiome. There have been found to be specific strains of bacteria that, if taken regularly for a few weeks, can lift depression and quell anxiety. Researchers Collins & Bercik stated that, "Bidirectional signaling between the gastrointestinal tract and the brain is thought to be mandatory for homeostasis, and integrates neural, hormonal, and immunological signaling." (*The interplay between the intestinal microbiota and the brain*, Nature Reviews Microbiology, 2012)

Some use the phrase, 'following your gut' instead of trying to weigh pros and cons with logic that may be minus insight. This phrase has some science behind it as a study by Pinilla states that, "*In addition to the capacity of the gut to directly stimulate molecular systems that are associated with synaptic plasticity and   learning, several gut hormones or peptides, such as leptin, ghrelin, (appetite regulators) glucagon-like peptide 1, and insulin have been found to influence emotions and cognitive processes.*"

These authors go further to state that, "*New studies showing that leptin promotes rapid changes in hippocampal dendritic morphology suggest that leptin exerts a direct action on hippocampal plasticity.*" (Fernando Gomez-Pinilla, "*Brain foods: the effects of nutrients on brain function*", Nature Reviews Neuroscience, July 2008). So the belly is in direct contact with several brain regions that can access memories, including relevant information about whatever's in front of you. In addition, recent studies have found that neuropod cells in the gut lining interface directly with the afferent fibers of the vagus nerve, reaching the brain in milliseconds with information from the intestines. This is much faster and more direct than the routes whereby hormones send information via the blood. (Marlek V. Bradford, "*Gut

Feelings are Hardwired", for Duke University, 2018) There are brain regions that make the decision for us about which stimuli will reach the part of consciousness that can perceive the stimuli, and which content will be filtered out. What is the basis of these 'parental control' buttons in the brain? Is it based upon prior interests, biases, genetics, or momentary relevance?

Logan and Katzman report that, *"Research states that bacteria in the GI tract can communicate with the central nervous system, even in the absence of an immune response. Probiotics have the potential to lower systemic inflammatory cytokines, decrease oxidative stress, improve nutritional status, and correct SIBO. The effect of probiotics on systemic inflammatory cytokines and oxidative stress may ultimately lead to increased brain derived factor (BDNF)."* (Major depressive disorder: probiotics may be an adjuvant therapy, National Institute of Health, 2005)

M. Hassan Mohajeri and his team go on to say that, *"It is now known that the benefits of human-microbe symbiosis can be extended to human mental health, and... the bi-directional communication between the resident microbes of the GI tract and the brain plays a key role in maintaining brain health. The GI microbiota influences human behavior and may affect the pathophysiology of mental illnesses."* (Mohajeri, et al, "Relationship between the gut microbiome and the brain; Oxford Academic nutrition Reviews, Vol. 76, Issue 7, July 2018)

Since the breakdown of social behavior is a common result of combat vets who have had baropressure brain injuries and seen in those ex-football players who died from CTE, probiotics may be a useful intervention following a concussion of any kind. Cognitive difficulties are also implicated in TBI, which can also be improved via the enteric nervous system, or our second brain in the belly. An article in Neurobiology of Stress states, *"The complex and multifaceted system of gut-brain communication not only ensures proper maintenance and coordination of gastrointestinal functions to support behavior and physiological processes, but also permits feedback from the gut to exert profound effects on mood, motivated behavior, and higher cognitive functions."* (Foster, Rinaman & Cryan, "Stress & the gut-brain axis: Regulation by the microbiome," Neurobiology of Stress, Vol. 7, December 2017.)

Kathleen Jade, in her article on "The Best Probiotics for Mood", describes the category of probiotics that can be helpful for depression as 'psychobiotics' which effect mood in three ways:
- Their ability to produce biological compounds like neurotransmitters such as GABA, serotonin, catecholamines, and acetylcholine, which, when secreted can trigger cells within the gut lining to release molecules that signal the brain
- They can help ameliorate consequences of the stress response and the presence

of cortisol in the system which "is believed to play a central role in causing mood disorders and cognitive problems.'

- They can act on inflammation, which can also come from the gut but can be present in the brain after injury

She lists those probiotics tested to help with depression as being Lactobacillus acidophilus, Lactobacillus casei, and Bifidobacterium bifidum. Not only were those who participated in this 8-week study reporting significantly less depression, but inflammatory markers were also down accompanied by a rise in the body's natural antioxidant, glutathione. Lactobacillus Helvetica may be helpful in reducing stress-related anxiety. (Kathleen Jade ND, *The Best Probiotics for Mood: Psychobiotics May Enhance the Gut-Brain Connection*, University Health News, June, 2018). Keep in mind that one result from taking antibiotics can be an imbalance in the microbiome, which can lead to a mood disorder and reduced protection.

In a separate study, Dr. Emily Deans observed a reduction in anxiety using lactobacillus rhamnosus on mice presumed to be related to its effect on the vagus nerve. (Emily Deans, MD, *"Do Probiotics Help Anxiety? More evidence on the gut-brain connection"*, Psychology Today, June, 2012) Bifidobacterium longum was previously known for its effect on depression, but has also been shown to help anxiety, obsessions, compulsions, and paranoia also through its influence on the vagus nerve. (Jordan Fallis, *"The 9 Most promising Psychobiotics for Anxiety"*, Optimal Living Dynamics, August, 2017) He also included Lactobacillus plantarum, Lactobacillus helveticus, Lactobacillus reuteri, Lactobacillus casei and a few others.

The heart-brain connection

The Netherlands Heart Journal published an article in 2013 that underscored the importance of modern medicine's less myopic view in the approach to resolving health issues. Author M.J. Daemen states, *"It is time for a more integrative view to the heart-brain connection as recent data indicates that cardiovascular conditions contribute to cognitive impairment."* Daemon goes on to cite that the growing appreciation between vascular risk factors and Alzheimer's disease could open doors to new protocols in the prevention of dementia. Noetic Systems International produced an article describing the flow of information in the form of afferent signs from the heart "have a regulatory influence on the autonomic nervous system, including most organs and glands", then goes on to say that, *"Cardiovascular afferents have numerous connections to the thalamus, hypothalamus, amygdala, which all play an important role in determining our perceptions, thought processes, and emotional experiences."* (Dr. D. Surel, *"Thinking from the heart; heart brain science"*, Edge Science Magazine, 2014).

Author Laura Saunders writes about the connection between the vascular and nervous system. *"New discoveries have shown a greater connection between the blood and the brain. In the new findings, it is evident that blood can actually control nerve cells. Alzheimer's disease is linked to 'dropped calls' between the blood and brain, creating 'silent patches' in the brain that affect how the brain is able to operate."* Apparently when the nerves need more fuel or oxygen, they signal the vessels to dilate and deliver more of the necessary nutrients, perhaps along the endothelial cells in the walls of the vessels, but when these cells are damaged due to mechanical or chemical injury, they can no longer function properly, depriving the brain of what it needs to survive. (Laura Sanders, analyzed by Jessica Vela, *"Blood Exerts a Powerful Influence on the Brain"*, Science News, 2015)

The microbiome of the belly also can have a powerful effect on the heart because it has an important role in the absorption, metabolism, and excretion of toxins, including heavy metals and environmental toxins, which are all implicated in heart disease. Since the guts are largely responsible for the availability of nutrients, if there is an imbalance in the belly's microbiome, the brain could also be deprived of certain nutrients like vitamin K and B vitamins that help the brain detox, as well as the inflammatory role played by the intestines that support the health of both the brain, the heart, and bones. The interplay between the heart, belly, and head brains renders them functionally interdependent. This interdependence is the basis for including that which serves the health of the heart and vascular system as well as the health of the gut to be thorough in approaching ways to recover from brain injuries.

Lymphatics and the Brain

There's been a lot of excitement in recent years about the discovery of the connection between the circulating cerebral spinal fluid in the brain and the lymphatic system. As long ago as 1899 Andrew T. Still, the father of Osteopathic Medicine, said, *"The lymphatics are closely and universally connected with the spinal cord and all other nerves, long or short, universal or separate, and all drink from the same waters of the brain."* There may have been a gap before the latter thoughts that described routing of the CSF via the choroid plexi in the lateral ventricles to the third, then down Sylvan's fissure to the 4th ventricle to the spinal cord and to the aperture of Lushka (that circulates around the brain) were updated.

Recent findings show that the lymphatic system is also connected to the small blood vessels in the brain's cerebral tissue, in that a great deal of lymph production happens there instead of mainly in the choroid plexi as previously thought. In the brain there is interstitial fluid, cerebrospinal fluid, and blood, which intersect one another. The role of the lymph in our bodies is to cleanse and filter waste and debris, like dead cells, from the system but it also contains immune cells that can kill microbes. The interstitial fluid in the brain is

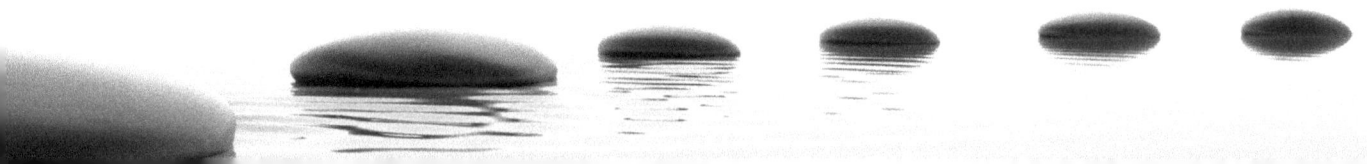

involved in cell-to-cell communication for drug delivery, distribution and clearance for brain ionic homeostasis, for immune function, clearance of beta-amyloid, and for the migration of cells.

Scientists from the University of Virginia observed lymph vessels in the central nervous system of the brain. They *"demonstrated that the lymphatic system extends into the dura mater, the thickest and outer-most of the three meningeal membranes that envelope the brain and spinal cord. These vessels run parallel to the major veins and arteries and split to send branches deep into the brain's crevices."* (Mo Costandi, *"How to Optimize Your Brain's Disposal System"*, August 2015) Other studies have found that there is an exit route through the cribiform plate and nasal mucosa through to the cervical lymph nodes.

Sun, Wang, et al report that, *"The brain lymphatic drainage system is composed of basement membrane-based perivascular pathways, a brain-wide glymphatic pathway, and cerebrospinal fluid drainage routes that include sinus-associated meningeal lymphatic vessels and olfactory/cervical lymphatic routes."* (*"Lymphatic drainage system of the brain: A novel target for intervention of neurological diseases"*, <u>Progressive Neurobiology</u>, May, 2018) A team of University researchers discovered how these fluids circulate the brain and expel waste after drilling a hole in the skull of mice and injecting a tracer dye.

The researchers observed that, *"like a river, cerebrospinal fluid carried these molecules rapidly along specific channels. Glial cells along the outside of arteries form these channels, creating a flume for cerebrospinal fluid that follows the brain's blood vessels. In addition, the researchers found that these glial cells mediate the channels' activity. From channels alongside arteries, the tracer-bearing fluid then passes through brain tissues. At the other end of tissues, it flows into similar channels along veins. The fluid follows these veins, then either returns to the subarachnoid space, enters the bloodstream, or eventually drains into the body's lymphatic system."* (Nedergaard et al, Science Translational Medicine, 2012)

Author and neuroscientist Jeff Iliff noted that one of the surprises in this study was the fact that the cycling of the fluid was a two-way, rather than one-way street as previously thought. The team saw that up to 40% of the CSF that carried waste material out of the brain into the body for removal was recycled back into the brain. The scientists later injected amyloid plaque proteins into the brains of two different groups of mice, one with normal brains, and one with a disabled glial cell system, and observed that the plaques were efficiently removed by the CSF in mice with normally functioning glial (astrocytes) cells. (Daisy Juhas, *"Brain Drain: Neuroscientists Discover Cranial Cleansing System, Fluids coursing through the brain could help clear the brain of toxic detritus that leads to Alzheimer's and Huntington's disorders"*, <u>Scientific American</u>, August 2012).

During a separate study in 2013, after wondering why beta-amyloid levels decreased at night, Nedergaard and her team of scientists injected the dye in the CSF of mice and tracked the flow of the dye again, and found very little activity during the day while it flowed freely during sleep or unconscious under anesthesia. The scientists also discovered that the extracellular space increased in volume by 60% while asleep or anesthetized, and that the amyloids disappeared twice as fast. The author of this article concludes by saying, "*The study raises the possibility that certain neurological disorders might be prevented or treated by manipulating the glymphatic system.*" (National Institutes of Health, October 2013)

Although sleep quality effects brain performance in just about everyone, it's particularly significant for aging adults as there is a consequential decrease in slow wave activity, the deeper sleep wave when working memory can be transformed into a stored memory. Hippocampal cells, which are most active for transforming short term to long term memory, are particularly vulnerable to die-off during trauma, but may also shrink with age. Sleep quality may well be a significant factor in the brain's ability to cleanse and restore itself, so could be an important area of continued investigation, particularly for trauma patients and seniors. To that end, Nedergaard and her team also discovered that side-sleeping produces better drainage for the brain than sleeping on the back.

Dr. Bruno Chikly states, "*It is exciting that the classical models of CSF physiology and the lymphatic anatomy in the CNS have both been dramatically updated with recent research. Our vision and understanding of lymphatics is profoundly expanded, giving us entry into deeper levels of healing, which now includes the brain. This new scientific evidence also opens the way for new manual techniques to arise that are more consistent with this evidence, giving the practitioner's work a higher level of credibility and acceptance in the health-care field.*"

Meditation and the Brain

Throughout the ages we've heard about the incredible feats accomplished by yogis who dedicate their lives to meditation and dietary changes that support their meditation practice. They've been able to gain control over many autonomic functions like breath, heartbeat, temperature, and some have even defied gravity through levitation. In modern times, some researchers have investigated the health benefits of Transcendental Meditation and found positive results. More recently researchers have discovered that not only can autonomic markers like blood pressure, heart rate, anxiety and stress be reduced, but brain changes also occur.

A study at UCLA found that "long-term meditators had better preserved brains than non-meditators as they aged". Twenty year veteran meditators had more grey matter and less volume loss compared to younger meditators or non-meditators. The researchers

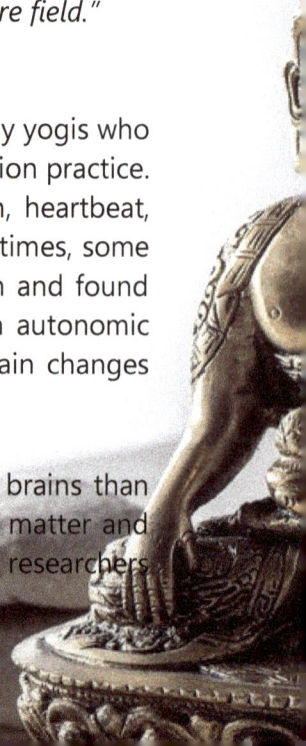

noticed a widespread effect encompassing several regions of the brain rather than more localized influences, although the Default Mode Network was one area that exhibited less activity. DMN activation represents a greater number of wandering thoughts, ruminating, and self-referential thoughts that are more common in people who aren't happy.

Just a few weeks of meditation has been shown to improve concentration and attention, memory, as well as improving mood and a sense of well-being. Jon Kabat-Zinn developed a form of meditation called Mindfulness-Based Stress Reduction which has been able to help people with anxiety even years after completing the 8-week course. Using this program also enabled people to overcome addictions. Another study in China involving a brief 5-day meditation practice was able to confirm greater conflict resolution, decrease in stress response, an increase in immune response, reduced anger, anxiety, depression and fatigue. Methods used were from Chinese medicine combining integrative body-mind training and mainly influenced the improvement in the executive attention network of the brain related to self-regulation. (Yi Yuan Tang, et al, *Proceedings of the National Academy of Sciences*, 2007).

Dr. Andrew Newbert from the University of Pennsylvania found that Tibetan Monks who meditated had their frontal lobes light up in a way that other brain wave studies confirm as a sign of high intelligence and faster levels of processing information in the high Beta or Gamma range. Also, while the parietal lobe that is connected to a sense of self heats up when loneliness is experienced, the same area is found to be cool in meditators who more often can have a sense of being connected to everything or everyone. A separate UCLA study in 2012 found that meditators have more balanced brains. The fibers in the corpus callosum which connects the two hemispheres in the brain were "remarkably stronger, thicker, and more connected in meditation practitioners".

This author goes on to state that, "Harmonizing the brain hemispheres opens the door to a smorgasbord of benefits, with better focus, deeper thought, super creativity, excellent mental health, enhanced memory, and clearer thinking..." Perhaps part of the reason that depression is decrease in meditators is because the brains of depressed people have considerable shrinkage in the hippocampus. Meditators have increased size and density of the hippocampus as well as the areas of the brain related to empathy and compassion. (Lutz, et al, PloS One, 2008). This is all to say the brain's plasticity and self-reformation can happen with someone as inexpensive and accessible as meditation.

Music and the Brain

In her 2014 article on the benefits of adults learning music, Sharon Bryant lists several benefits for the brain cited by researchers. Some include enhanced perception of speech,

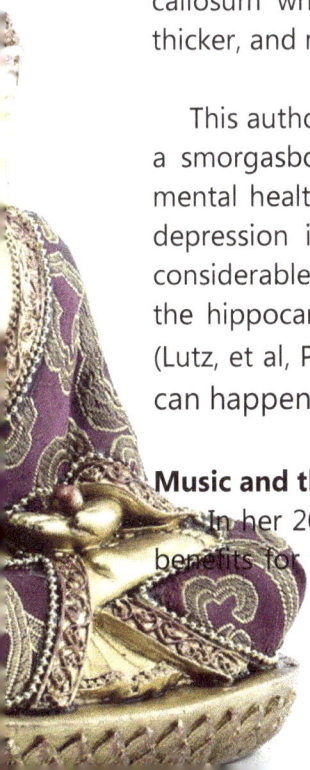

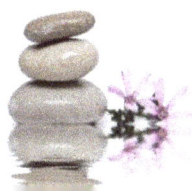

more proficient auditory working memory, and auditory attention. (Annals of the New York Academy of Sciences, 2015). Apparently music "engages the part of the brain involved with paying attention, making predictions, and updating events in working memory." (Stanford Medicine, 2015) She also cites Berti et al., 2006 who found that musicians have a superior working memory compared to non-musicians. Somehow, those with fairly advanced dementia or Alzheimer's do become more alert and responsive when listening to familiar music.

Neuromusicology is a branch of science dedicated to the study of the brain as it relates to processing music, whether playing or listening to it. As music has been used as a therapeutic approach for generations, more attention has been drawn to music recently on how to best use its influence. The results of a study published in Nature Neuroscience found that the brains of musicians are larger and more sensitive than non-musicians while Gaser and Schlaug showed that brain centers responsible for motor control, auditory processing, and spatial coordination are also larger in musicians. (Journal of Neuroscience, October 2003) Similar to the findings for meditators, they also have larger corpus callosums where information is passed between the left and right hemispheres of the brain.

Singers are also reported to have brains that are different than non-singers. As a whole, they are fitter, happier and more productive, have fewer stress hormones in their systems with more oxytocin - the hormone that stimulates bonding and happiness. Singing also produces higher levels of immunoglobulin A, which is responsible for health of the respiratory and digestive tracts. The breathing required by professional singers promotes cardiovascular health, while they can also exhibit better working memory, and higher activation of the basal ganglia, thalamus, cerebellum and prefrontal cortex regions related to goal-directed attention. (Kleber et al, *Cerebral Cortex*, May 2010). Even amateur singers experience many of the emotional and cognitive benefits of singing, especially when singing with a group, but even if singing alone in the shower positive changes happen.

Taxi drivers also exhibit specific brain changes because they're continually developing additional spatial orientation skills, which is to say that most activities entered into on a regular basis. It is ever responsive and adapting to our use patterns. It retains plasticity as long as we are alive and continuing to explore new options, or developing increased awareness within what we are already engaged in. "Use it or lose it" applies to the brain as well as to muscle power, so by continuing to challenge it and awaken those pathways to new information can lead to a much longer, healthier, and happier life. The brain rewires itself according to how and how often you use it. I mentioned the effect of meditation and music on the brain not only to point out the diverse, marvelously complex, responsive, and vastness of the brain's many capacities, but also because spending 40 years singing regularly and 30 years using some form of mediation regularly may have made it possible to function okay the first forty years with my head injuries and still be able to function and still rebound after another 25 years of injury. (Knock on wood.)

The enigmatic right brain

Jill Bolte-Taylor gained widespread attention when she, as a neurologist, was fascinated by her brain's journey after she had a fairly major stroke on the left side of her brain at 37 years old. She'd made mental notes during the entire process of her limited ability to reach a phone and find someone to call as her brain function was rapidly declining. What was even more fascinating to Dr. Taylor was being able to watch her brain switch to the right hemisphere,

LEFT HEMISPHERE

- Responsible for logical thinking
- Focused in analysis
- Responsible for language skills
- Controls speech
- Responsible for memorizing facts and names
- Controls reading and writing abilities
- Controls science and mathematical capabilities
- Specializes in sequential processing of information
- Controls right part of the body

RIGHT HEMISPHERE

- Focused in intuition
- Conceives the non-verbal information
- Responsible for spatial orientation
- Focused in synthesis
- Responsible for ability to draw pictures
- Responsible for imagination
- Responsible for musicality
- Creates emotions
- Produces dreams
- Specializes in multitasking and parallel processing of information
- Controls left part of the body

all reported with detail in her book on the subject called, "Stroke of Insight", which was published in 2008.

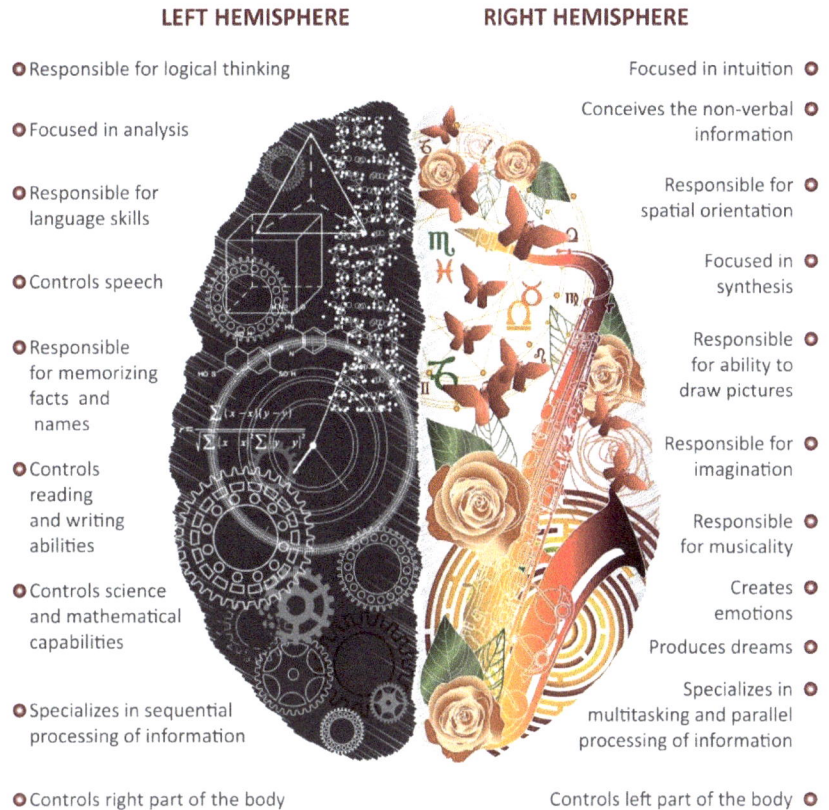

She was excited to experience calm and a vast, euphoric peace in her right brain although she'd lost the ability to walk, read, or speak and could barely dial the phone for help. On the other hand, Dr. Brick Johnstone found that 20 patients with damage to the right parietal lobe reported more incidences of transcendental experiences. (Johnstone, Bodling, et al, *"Right Parietal Lobe-Related Selflessness as the Neurophysiological Basis of Spiritual Transcendence"*, The International Journal for the Psychology of Religion, Vol. 22, 2012). Seemingly where impressions related to selfhood are stored, this same region has diminished in meditators who report mystical or spiritual experiences beyond the body-mind-ego. Religious practices like prayer, however, light up the frontal lobe. Author Santoro reports that centuries ago, Leonardo da Vinci placed the soul above the optic chiasm in the region of the anterior-inferior third ventricle and that possibly da Vinci was the first person to accurately locate this chiasm. I can attest that the third ventricle, being an area of focus in Biodynamic Cranial work, not only feels special but elicits a sublime nectar that is related to an esoteric aspect of the heart.

Dr. Jealous expressed wisdom from Rollin Becker about the Tide within the Biodynamic process as such: *"A little knowledge creates projections... Knowledge from the Tide creates love. Knowledge begins with our education. Later, as the Tide heals us, we come to know being love beyond our belief. All our knowledge will die in the movement of the healing in ourselves. There is direct knowledge from the Tide that comes with us at conception and stays with us throughout life. Osteopathy is from and about that knowledge."* (James Jealous, D.O., An Osteopathic Odyssey, 2015) The forefathers and many practitioners of this body of work carry a most wonderful, honoring and respectful approach to the system's ability to heal itself when connected to its inner Divinity, all the while delicately and very specifically addressing the structures that facilitate and/or inhibit the flow of that current.

We seem to need science along the way to convince the mind of what the heart already has the ability to know directly, and even the most Ancient practices are not without scientific study and validation. Dr. Andrew Newberg scanned the brains of Buddhists and nuns during mystical experiences "reporting feelings of timelessness, spacelessness, and self-transcendence" and also saw reduced activity in the parietal lobe where the brain interprets the relationship between the body and objects in space (exteroceptors) as well as the relationship between parts of one's own body (interoceptors). In one case a person with damage in this area didn't believe his leg was his own and tried to get it out of the bed. In more extreme cases patients request that a limb be amputated. (Andrew Newberg M.D., *"The Metaphysical Mind: Probing the Biology of Philosophical Thought"*, 2013).

Lisa Miller and her team suspects that those who've had a variety of spiritual experiences may also have corresponding brain changes. It makes sense that if it remodels according to every other activity a person is frequently engaged in, why wouldn't the same be true for meditation, Grace, and other sources of spiritual experiences? Perhaps instead of those experiences being found or produced there, the brain modifies those circuits accordingly, storing them as such, so each additional experience strengthens those pathways and makes the state easier to access. Miller observed reduced activity in the inferior parietal lobe during guided imagery involving meaningful spiritual experiences, as well as reduced activity in the medial thalamus and caudate nucleus, "regions associated with sensory and emotional processing". This was observed in people who were not having spiritual experiences, but were imagining them, yet the same areas were lighting up as the memories were being triggered. Miller, Balodis, et. al., *"The Neural Correlates of Personalized Spiritual Experiences,"* Cerebral Cortex, May 2018).

Those who have spiritual experiences out of the context of a teacher can be very confused for a while as there's no frame of reference for what happened. Many if not most enlightened teachers report of expanded experiences while being still a toddler if not early on in elementary school, only to have the space open up again as a young adult and remain permanent. Some have even seen an image of their future teacher at 3 or 4 years old and were surprised to be drawn to a place where they would meet that teacher in person decades later. I heard many such stories while living in India. A well-known Advaita teacher, Robert Adams, was one who saw Ramana Maharshi by his crib when he was a toddler.

We commonly think of the right brain as being the creative hemisphere where some say writers, musicians, dancers, and artists draw their inspiration, talent, and abilities from as well as where intuition lives. Jan Engels –Smith in her blog, *"Being in Your Right Brain"*, describes it as the place where we process non-verbal stimuli and more holistic, as opposed to linear thinking. Apparently though, when the dysfunction happens early enough, the brain can make remarkable adaptations so the person can lead a normal life without portions of their brain. Children with debilitating seizures have undergone successful surgeries to remove either the right or left hemisphere of the brain, then went on to graduate from college.

In one unusual case, a man with only 10% of his brain left led a normal life in relatively good health with a job, wife, and two children. He'd had hydrocephalus as a child whereby there was a fluid build-up that had been largely removed by a stent. But after complaining of slight weakness in his leg, the doctors discovered that over the 30 years since the stent had been removed at age 14, the majority of his brain had eroded. The author of this article states, *"Not only did his case study cause scientists to question what it takes to survive, it also challenges our understanding of consciousness"*. (Fiona Macdonald, *"Meet the Man Who Lives Normally with Damage to 90% of His Brain,"* Science Alert Magazine, July 2016)

Stanislaus Dehaene, in his article, *"The Brain Mechanisms of Conscious Access and Introspection"*, considers certain aspects of consciousness, including the ability to bring thoughts to the forefront of awareness, as being a characteristic of being human. Other creatures can also certainly do the same thing, as well as make enough distinctions to be able to learn from their environment and experiences. But Deheane then cites Vladimir Nabokov who says, *"Being aware of being aware of being... if I not only know that I am but also know that I know it, then I belong to the human species."*

Consciousness and thought

Dehaene goes on to say that *"Philosophical approaches failed to shed much light on the problem of how an assembly of nerve cells could produce conscious thoughts."* There are not only thoughts, but there is also a 'thinker', the one to whom perceptions appear. Some are still trying to locate that one by the region of the brain that becomes activated when thoughts or emotions occur, or when self-referencing happens. There is someone who can be aware of awareness and of self-reflection, or of the body's, the mind's, and the ego's activities in a way that liberates that 'one' from those activities and thoughts. Buddha has called thought the smallest particle of consciousness.

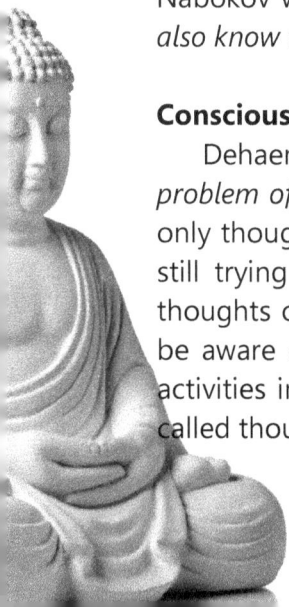

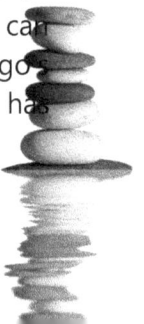

Buddha is reported to have said, "All things are preceded by the mind, led by the mind, created by the mind." This teaching separates the mind from mental factors in terms of form, but not in terms of function. Buddhism says, "*Whenever we see the kin (consciousness) we see the servants (mental factors). When mind arises and cognizes an object, it is accompanied by several mental factors that help the mind in cognizing the object.*"

Buddhism believes that *'There is no permanent entity as a person. It is merely a name for a combination of elements. They include body, feeling perception, mental formation and consciousness. We think of ourselves as having a permanent identity or 'I' because we identify with the moment-to-moment processes of changing phenomena'*. (Global Buddhist Door, October 2013). The cetasikas are those that give color to the Cittas (the awareness of the object that is being perceived) which can arise as being beautiful, as being neutral, or as unwholesome Cittas.

The Cittas (consciousness) and cetasikas arise together and are dependent upon one another. Cetasikas, vidhis, and citta are described in great detail in the Abhidhamma, a part of an ancient Theravada Buddhist text that has over 6000 pages in its comprehensive description of how the mind functions. According to professors, Barendregt & Mulder in their body of work, *"Interpreting the Abhidhamma: ingredients of consciousness"*, there is no continuity in consciousness, but only flashes, or consciousness moments strung together by their inherent components. The concepts that string them together are called ceta (or citta), cetasika, and vithi. Cetas are flashes of consciousness or 'mind-moments' that come in sequences that could be called thoughts. Their actions are divided into arising, (presence) performing its momentary function, and dissolution – just like the sub-quarks. These authors go on to say that the speed of these events is so fast that they are seen as one continuous action. The cetas are directed towards the content of consciousness, an object, i.e. something perceived by the senses, to which it becomes attached - like the interpretation, attitude, or belief about the object.

Depending upon how the objects or content of consciousness are viewed, either with positive (wholesome), negative (unwholesome), or neutral cetasikas, the future cetasikas are then bound by their respective positive or negative karmas or consequences. Attraction or repulsion based upon the interpretation of the object that might be associated with thoughts of desire or hatred, anger, etc. can also be binding. Most spiritual teachers will either advise aspirants to meditate upon the space between thoughts, or to aim towards a neutral disposition with whatever arises - thoughts within, or objects without. Most religions guide parishioners towards wholesome thoughts or wholesome interpretations of events.

Wholesome (or beautiful) attitudes are seen to be able to decondition unwholesome ones, and eventually free a person from negative karma or consequences of the more

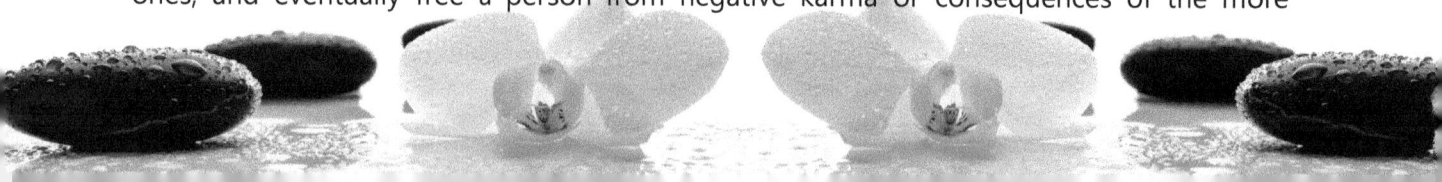

negative reactions. Part of the aim of Buddhism is to ease human suffering, which these teachings can do. There are 89 types of cetas which will not be listed here, but it can be useful to hear that these types are divided into planes. There are three planes that include the sensual, the sublime, and the supramundane planes. The sensual pertains to daily life sensory input and the preference for that input to be pleasant; the sublime refers to exalted mystical states, and the supramundane exhibits purified consciousness that is devoid of certain types of cetas.

This branch of Buddhism observes the presence of a baseline of citta - of consciousness - that is continuous. Some paths may call this the ground of being, others may call it the screen upon which perceptions and thoughts appear. Vithis, in this tradition, are cognitive/emotional factors that appear like a stream of thoughts, sequences of cetas. There have been 17 sensory and 12 mental vithis delineated that have phases of the sensory input or thought arising, then being pulled from memory, named, then assigned meaning. These vithis gain power based upon the meaning given to them.

Although it seems like a lot to digest, these are moment-to-moment processes in the brain that happen automatically and drive, if not control the personality and the person. The baseline consciousness or ground of being, the space between thoughts can be seen as analogous to a stem cell ceta. It is an unprogrammed or unconditioned aspect of consciousness that is free and can support the reorganization and balance of those cells that have unhealthy ideas or pain patterns attached to them. It is a way that consciousness can be employed as a form of treatment by shifting into another plane that can be the bridge for unhealthy patterns to be released against a neutral, empty screen.

In this case, and in most cases with Eastern Spirituality, the truth of who we really are is the vast, timeless, (supramundane) Universal Self that is one with our consciousness, with all of life, but that is also the indweller of the body, mind, and brain. Most of Eastern spirituality guides its practitioners towards neutral witnessing of the objects that appear in front of this screen of consciousness, while adding that the observer and the observed are one, but who we are is neither. We are the primordial Source from which both arise. Kundalini yoga is one process that helps to awaken and encourage the Shakti at the base of the spine to move up through all the restrictions (as life experiences or karmas) in the nadis and chakras up to the crown where one it's possible to realize the Godhead. Although purported to be a very long path that can even take lifetimes, meditation and yoga are meant to help clear all the many 'obstructions' along these pathways that restrict the flow of Shakti.

Along the way many subtle phenomena can arise and even supra-mental abilities or 'siddhis' as they can be called, as the limitations to what 'super' consciousness is cable of are

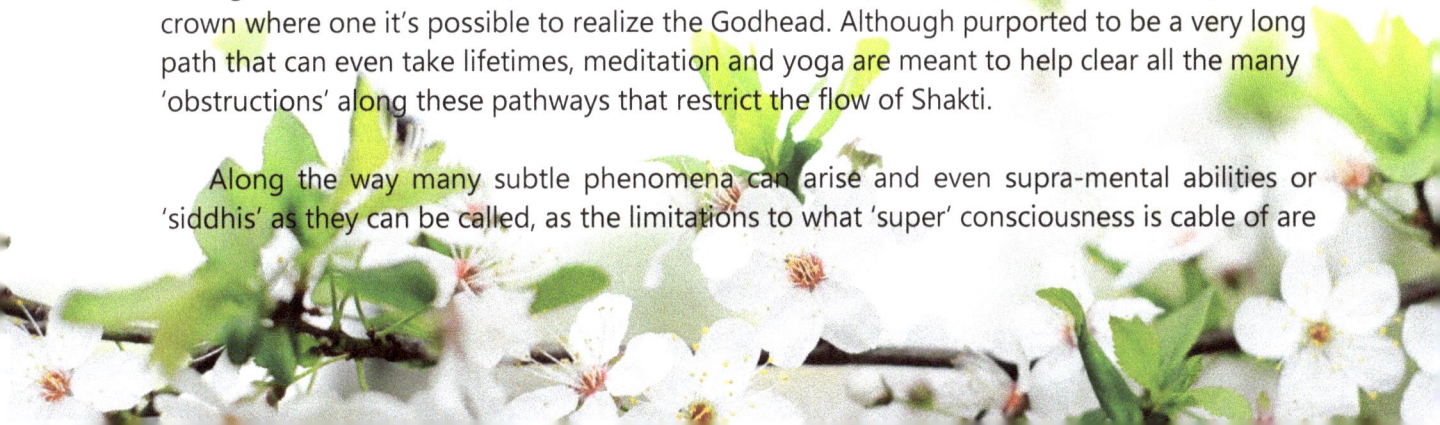

removed. These so-called obstructions or restrictions are none other than traumas or memories that we identify with that have captured our attention and retained our focus on life's ups and downs. Those 'restrictions' to the flow of Shakti near the spinal cord may also limit one's ability to be aware of the potential of consciousness. Yet exhilarating and awful experiences create an impression on the brain because our neurophysiology compels them to, and it's a slippery slope to ignore pain when the body's putting out a warning of harm.

Probably 99% of spiritual and religious practices are on how to be with those challenges in the most optimal way, according to the faith, belief, or direct experience in the Higher Power. Good health and longevity in general, do change the brain, along with its neurotransmitters, and promote a happier existence. Prayer - as a form of thought - has been known to produce miracles, including bringing loved ones back to life after being pronounced dead. In 2006, Dr. Chauncey Crandall was able to bring a heart attack patient back to life after all post-surgical attempts to revive him failed by praying for him. This man was already in the morgue when the cardiologist heard a voice ask him to return to the man and pray for him. The doctor finally complied, returned to the deceased, and asked for his life to be returned in the name of God.

In another remarkable incident in Africa, a small asthmatic boy who died of tuberculosis was revived by prayer after many people in the village he lived in participated in a group prayer. When he returned to visit the doctor who had pronounced him dead, not only was he alive and well, but the asthma was gone. These incidents aren't rare, but can be confusing when a loved one isn't healed, or when one doesn't feel heard in an hour of need. If the brain has quadrillions of connections that are much too complex to comprehend, imagine how complex and difficult it is to comprehend the Universe and its consciousness.

Larry Dossey in his article entitled, "Why the Brain is not Consciousness", states that *"Consciousness can operate beyond the brain, body and the present, as hundreds of experiments and millions of testimonials confirm. Consciousness, therefore, cannot be identical with the brain."* Countless people have 'arisen' from their bodies while under anesthesia and reported with great detail and accuracy what they saw in the operating room during their surgical procedures. They could all verify Dossey's statement. Did the surgery patients suddenly achieve that state of global awareness like what spontaneously happened to me in India – being able to see with something other than physical eyes? There's nothing like a life-or-death urgency to wake up consciousness or special feats.

Belief, faith, intent, emotions, and thoughts can all influence consciousness, physiology, and neurophysiology, but what consciousness is lies beyond all of them. Cell biologist, Dr. Bruce Lipton, has shown that receptor sites can change their shape to open to a ligand that would otherwise not be drawn to bind there based solely upon belief. So far, in many instances the effects of thoughts and feelings have been observed without having seen an actual thought. Candace Pert was able to identify specific proteins/ligands that were activated with the expression of emotions, however I'm not sure that we can say that emotion is synonymous with a protein. Science by its nature needs to reduce complex human experiences into something predictable, observable, and measurable. Consciousness may not comply with this need.

This larger field of consciousness is so vast and so mysterious, it may manifest differently for you than for someone else. This intelligent field of awareness can be brought to bear on whatever symptom is arising from an injury and can participate in helping to bring the system back into balance. Some of the energetic qualities of the universal field can be experienced through the area near the optic chiasm in the brain, or through the heart, or dan tien - a couple of inches below the navel in the body's center of gravity. These are all common areas of focus in certain types of meditation practices.

In case the subject of consciousness is new to some readers, I'd like to offer a little background from different perspectives before exploring how aspects of consciousness can help in healing. It was far from being the only factor in my recovery, but one could say it had a fundamental role to play, regardless of the form of treatment. During the process of researching the subject of traumatic brain injury and the many ways it can rejuvenate and repair itself, I've realized that certain choices made may have unwittingly played a part in reducing the severity or tenacity of my symptoms. As many of you may have already found out or may also discover, it took years for me to realize that early injuries were still impacting my daily life.

It was only after a bad fall that rearranged the back of my skull that my body didn't bounce back the way it used to. I'd used up my 'reserves' so to speak, and the symptoms were extreme, prolonged, and unmissable. It then began to dawn on me that the earlier hits had a cumulative effect. The new symptoms were different from earlier ones that lived in a closed closet of unclarity, all the while screaming of error messages that finally couldn't be overlooked. It was clear that sustained intervention was going to be needed to get to the other side of that accumulation so that my system could build up reserves again and regain the capacity to adapt and to heal. Having been involved with sensory awareness and meditation for a while, the baseline – although itself not entirely normal – still enabled the newly introduced symptoms to stand out like lightning and thunder in the night sky.

Deciding to make use of the many sleepless nights the game-changing concussion supplied, I contemplated its symptoms against the substrate of consciousness and in the process learned a great deal about head injuries as well as about pain. Many, many times sitting in the substrate either greatly reduced or eliminated pain. It reminds me of the long

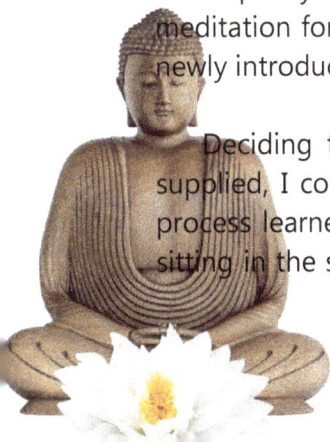

tide in Biodynamic Cranial work vs. the CRI layer of the body which has a faster rhythm and is where the physical, emotional, mental, and physiological attributes reside. The long tide, on the other hand, is where inherent health and its organizing principle live. In the long tide, there is only deep peace and restful calm.

It was during these daily contemplations that spanned over 15 years that the questions arose about what the form of 'thought' was. It must have some form to be able to influence as many systems (and people) as it does. It can't be formless. I searched high and low for literature from others who may have questioned what constitutes thought, but only Buddha himself covered it in detail. I became interested in the subject because I felt many times that what was vibrating in the field around and inside my body might be unassigned particles or undigested impressions from experiences that created tensions or restrictions.

These particles also engage the corpus callosum, dura, frontalis, temporalis, jaws, sub-occipitals, eyes, erectors, and trapezius muscles. I don't doubt that there are other areas, but these are the ones that stand out the most in my system. This is why it helps so much to try and notice the space between thoughts, which can be like trying to slip in between rain drops, but it's actually not that hard once you get used to it. It helps to envision the huge sky the rain is falling through rather than trying to dodge them; or in the same vein, to just envision the space the thoughts arise within. Countless nights, when contemplating and releasing these incoherent vibrations in and around my body, the spine and joints opened, tissue fields lengthened and softened, the mind and brain quieted, and soreness abated.

Some spiritual teachers compare thoughts to a wild horse that can take you on quite an adventurous if not dangerous ride if you can't rein them in. They shape our perceptions of the past and hopes for the future. They are the scaffolding for the present moment to rest upon, the bridge to the next moment, and are the basis for the tone of each day of our lives. They ebb and flow the waters of our sickness as well as our health, of our interactions with ourselves and with others, so why aren't science, cognitive neuroscience, psychiatry, psychology, biochemistry, and medicine in a queue in front of a microscope trying to find one and track it's interactions like Candace Pert did with emotions?

I guarantee that when researchers do locate the form of thoughts and observe them, they'll be found interfacing with every single molecule of our bodies and brains, like water and air. They will be found to be just as fundamental as any amino acid, lipid, neurotransmitter, hormone, or gene transcription factor whose character has as much of a role to play in regulating efficacy of function as the shaping of form. They will be seen as guardians who are just as important as the blood brain barrier, or anti-oxidants, or probiotics. They'll be recognized as gate-keepers for the flow of energy, of fluids, and of all the nano substances that nourish us from the womb forward. Thoughts are an intricate part

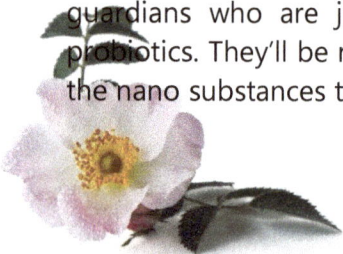

of every web of connective tissue, fluid, and network of communication that happens in the body. In a certain way, genetic coding is a form of thought, and thought is a form of coding.

Drs. Barral and Croibier mention that due to the law of conservation of energy, undissipated forces from accidents and falls can settle into fluids, fascia, and other systems, changing their fluid nature to a gel-like consistency, or an easily gliding fascial system into a dense, gummy one. These memories and impressions, like Dr. Wonderly's and The Abhidhamma's concepts suggest, can be tied into the system with the initial sensory impressions, their feeling states, with the attitude or belief about the experience, with similar memories from the past, as well as with the bio-mechanical forces that are present.

For example, a client who'd had chronic back and shoulder pain for years came into the Somatics clinic for a treatment. During the session it was revealed that she'd been attacked from behind on that side of her body and she hadn't made the connection until that moment. That was the glue that held that entire syndrome in her tissue field, and once it was realized at the same time the muscles were opening, there was reorganization of the field and it was able to discharge from her bodymind and not return. If there had been a family history of abuse or some other predisposition also associated with that event, it may have been a more complex web to unravel, but in her case, it was a one-and-done situation. Nonetheless, that spot in her shoulder had bothered her for many years without her making the connection to that emotional piece of the web.

Anyone can benefit from methods that help to reorganize traumatic injuries by touching into something that is a little more subtle than the layer where the injury or trauma sits. If you do believe that subtle, subconscious fields of influence can be in part contributing to the longevity or severity of your symptoms, even better. In either case, you're invited to walk with me through this labyrinth while I gradually unpack how I overcame a lifelong pattern of traumatic injury. In many instances, the injuries were the doors to ongoing awakening.

In the next chapter more detail will be given about which activities, practices, and treatments made it possible to recover so well (knock on wood). I'll also explore how in my case, developing one area of consciousness greatly benefitted another area and supported a type of lasting freedom. Alongside suggestions for choosing a healing protocol for an injured brain, I will also include specific remedies for the exacerbated symptoms that manifested in my bowling game. My body had adapted to all my other weekly activities, so without trying something new, I may never have been able to connect the dots between the unresolved, undiscovered residuals that were sitting in various layers of my system making exacerbation possible. The discoveries made in search of the source of those residuals were life-altering.

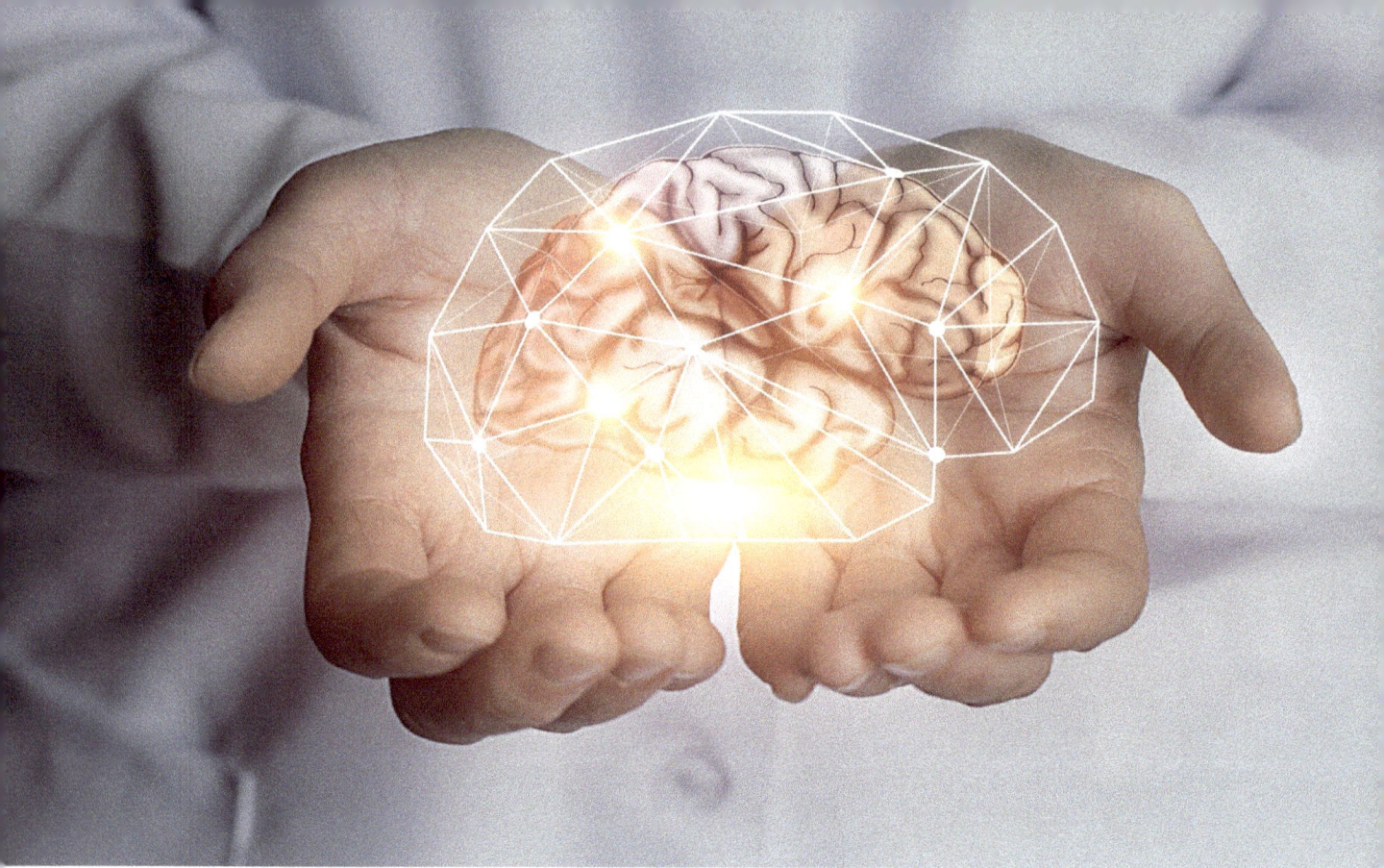

Chapter 4

Treating the Chicken and the Egg

*"Your body is precious. It is our vehicle for awakening.
Treat it with care."*

~Buddha

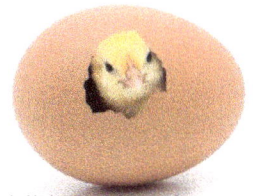

Did the egg benefit the chicken?

Looking back now it's so much easier to see that most of what created additional head injuries were those prior head injuries and the lack of information available about what to do about them to rebalance and restore my system, yet somehow I was able to maintain. Grave concerns were building due to the symptoms I was experiencing about 15 years before any of this research had hit mainstream. There were several lucky interventions along the way before the 'table-turning' catastrophic impacts that motivated me to seek medical help. These synchronistic events truly served my belief in miracles and serendipity.

Only in looking back can I see that some of the life choices and seeds planted along the way benefitted my orientation and familiarity with the territory of recovering from trauma. Someone without a history in holistic health could easily have felt lost or overwhelmed about where to start; that's another reason to write this book. Even in how to discern or differentiate which symptoms related to which trauma and how to find a practitioner or modality that matched the imbalance could be boggling without a little guidance. Hopefully the details listed here will resonate in a way that can demystify some of the many options out there so you can find the right fit for your system without feeling like you need to become a practitioner. Hopefully you can also save some money using self-treating options.

These days you can look on the internet and do a quick search that will pull up some great ideas and new treatment options for concussions and head trauma. However, if you're not familiar with the jargon being used or you're not sure how to connect the symptom with the technique, you might get some help from the journey I took to discover those very things. There are so many different types of pain and dysfunction that can happen during an acute phase of trauma and in the post-concussive phases that aren't common knowledge that family medicine practitioners may not be able to guide you with. Because I'd been searching for answers since my days as a school psychologist, I'd tried just about everything I could find that seemed like it could get to the bottom of neurological issues.

After a little investigating it became obvious that many of those school referrals sprang from emotional or physical trauma. School systems are not set up to deal with that, and neither are colleges, work places, and many doctors' offices. Unless you've broken or sprained, cut, or burned something, trauma outside of pharmaceutical intervention is a huge grey area for modern medicine. The fact that emotional, physiological, physical and performance issues could arise out of neurological ones is now more common knowledge. It can also be said now, that there are several complimentary disciplines that can help a lot with both diagnosis and treatment.

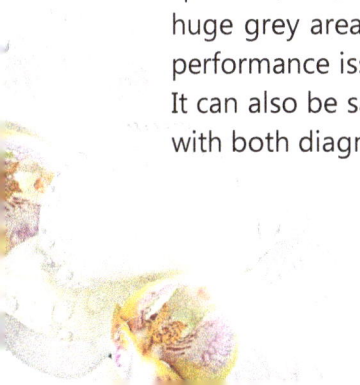

This key is worth mentioning more than once. **Tip #1**: Once you suspect that the symptoms might be related to brain injury, it's super important to seek care right away. Remember that it may take years for the damage to take a heavy toll and reveal itself fully. A recent study by biologists Gomez-Pinilla and Yang from UCLA reveals that the cell and gene damage from brain injuries can lead to brain disorders like Alzheimer's, Parkinson's, PTSD, and others. They discovered that *"hundreds of genes are adversely affected my mild, traumatic brain injury"*, including those that *"regulate metabolism, control thyroid hormones, and perform other functions"*. A promising result of the study was that by injecting T4 hormone into mice with head trauma, learning and memory deficits from damage to 93 genes related to brain injury were reversed. (Stuart Wolpert, *"UCLA cell study reveals how head injuries lead to serious brain diseases,* November 2018)

Like shingles sitting as a seed of possibility if you've had chicken pox as a child, dementia, personality disorders, CTE and other cognitive deficits can lie in the bushes waiting for you to be more vulnerable in middle age before jumping out to ambush your consciousness. Remember that in my case the brain fog had set in already, so I was lucky to have seeds and fertilizer that led me to head in the direction toward a more conscious life. It was the pull to a more conscious life that helped me shake the numbing fog and meet people who recommended processes that wound up healing body and mind. Along the way, the shifts in consciousness proved to be a tremendous resource that at times even felt magical.

The story will need to back up a little bit to tie the string of magic together more fully. My back had begun to heal and stabilize from those early missteps, but it was still a little fragile. After re-injuring myself dozens of times by refusing to accept the limits of the disc injury, I finally vowed to absolutely avoid the no-no's and take better care. I didn't sit down for almost seven years except to drive my car, and even then I pushed my back up against the seat so my butt didn't have to touch the seat. I used a wedge with a hole in it so if I did touch down there'd be minimal pressure on my sacrum. I learned from this earlier bout with a debilitating situation, but still had a ways to go. **Tip# 2:** at a significant cost, don't do things that can re-injure or trigger the trauma while it's healing. It cuts the healing time by months if not years.

During my first trip to northern India something amazing happened. Up until then, it had been virtually impossible for me to sit on a hard surface. If I ever let my butt sit on a surface, it had to be well cushioned and super comfy with plenty of leg room so I could change position when needed. Where I wound up in this case was in the living room of an enlightened Master, who I was super excited to meet. His name was H.W.L. Poonja, endearingly called Papaji. No one really knew how old he was, but the rumor was that he was already in his eighties and one should not delay to visit.

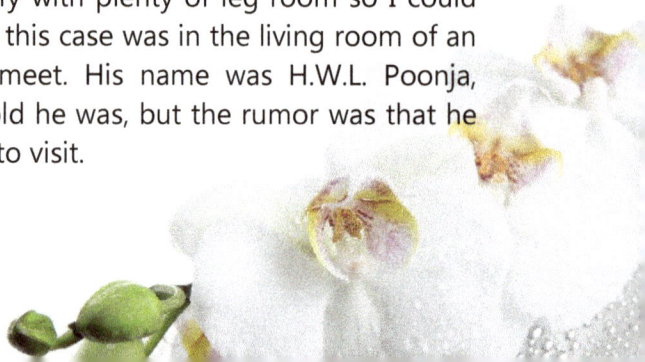

The setting was small and intimate, with a few dozen people in his living room when I first arrived. Within a month there were seventy-five people in a room that was about 10' x 12' with tile & cement floors. The cushions were raw cotton that didn't offer padding, and there wasn't room for very many, so most had to sit on their scarves or shawls. We couldn't sit cross-legged due to the number of people squeezed in, so we had to hug our knees in front of us to save space. At some point I realized that my back didn't hurt, and that there wasn't any pain or discomfort anywhere. After the twenty-four plus hours of plane rides, lay overs, with a six hour train ride, plus jet lag, I was stumped at how that was possible.

Something had transpired my first day there that had transformed everything in sight into a thing of beauty. Every pig, every mud pit, every pile of trash and 'road apple' seemed to glow and exude the same beauty. And on top of it, there was an incredible stillness that felt vast and beyond the goings on in the body or mind. In fact, not much at all was going on in the mind in terms of thoughts, and I wasn't as much aware of my brain as I was aware of my heart. The fullness that had arrived in the heart had superseded any discomfort in my body, which seemed to have gained a new levity and spaciousness.

This sudden shift in my perception left a lasting impression, because from then on I knew that there was a state whereby the body and mind could come to such a complete rest that there would be no discomfort or pain. I wasn't exactly certain if everything was magically healed, or if there was a particular way that the mind or brain had previously been engaging with the experience that was keeping it in play. In any case, I was certainly enjoying the freedom. This experience was very different than meditation. It was a different state of consciousness. I couldn't have gotten there through meditation, although being near Papaji did make meditation much easier and more absorptive.

It was beginning to sink in that my back did a little better with more protein, perhaps because dairy and eggs were out of the picture for me since the last time I lived in India. My digestion was much better, but the weakness that had come from being so restricted for so long required an occasional trip to town for tandoori chicken. I was pretty much in a state of bliss all the time after that experience, at the Grace of Papaji. My mind was quiet, my brain was still, I slept like a baby, and all was well as long as I had a little chicken and fish in my diet. **Tip #3**: Investigate possible dietary needs that support healing.

As soon as I'd felt strong enough and saved enough money, I was back on a plane to India. During one visit, a group of us went to Tiruvannamalai in Tamil Nadu near Madras in South India. While meditating in Virupaksha cave where Ramana Maharshi sat in silence for 17 years, my mind completely disappeared for about three weeks. I'd heard of the state of no-mind (mu shin) they'd often talked about in martial arts but had never really experienced it. Living from there was literally mind-blowing. The calm came from the mind not activating the personality or the body with emotion or reactions of any kind. Things were just as they were - thatāta - just as the senses perceived them and nothing more. **Tip #4**: Consider embracing a neutral disposition to your symptoms and life experiences wherever possible; it restores calm, dissipates trauma, and reveals more while facilitating clarity.

This again was quite different than the gap or blank-out that comes with a concussion, because in that tathāta state you're fully present taking everything in, but not doing anything with what comes in. The brain was at rest and not agitated in any way. There was a new kind of peace in this space; a kind where the goings on in daily life don't bother you at all, because they aren't processed through a personal memory or filter. The Grace of Arunachala had opened yet another door in consciousness that also bore subtle differences to the prior state of the mind falling into the heart. I believe that the time spent in these different layers of consciousness had shifted my overall perspective on life events, adding to the treasure chest of resources that benefitted the upcoming challenges.

What else can serve as a resource?

In my efforts to understand the traumas and health issues of my family, my students, and myself, I subjected myself to many therapeutic explorations. The first was Primal (Scream) Therapy in New York, which was like letting the pressure off of a steam cooker. I then studied Breath Therapy in India which was meant to super-charge the system with oxygen and support the body's release process, which felt fantastic. Several active meditations were at the ready from Bhagwan that you could either do in a group, or by yourself following the music on a tape. (In those days we used tapes, not CD's, mp3's, or ipods yet.)

- Dynamic Meditation happened early on, which had a few stages to it that included methods to discharge stress, a way to release neurotic or crazed impulses through sound and movement, a period of self-inquiry, and finally a stage to sit silently
- Kundalini meditation was a favorite, which mostly involved shaking tensions out of the body for a while before sitting quietly, and
- Nadabrahma meditation was also wonderful. This one had us sitting while circling our hands out for several minutes to 'exhale' all the bad stuff, then circle the hands inward to bring in the good stuff from the Universe
- Latihan was a way to allow the body to move itself in ways that it only knew in order to unwind restrictions. What a pleasant surprise to see the body energy take off and move itself with you just allowing the movement

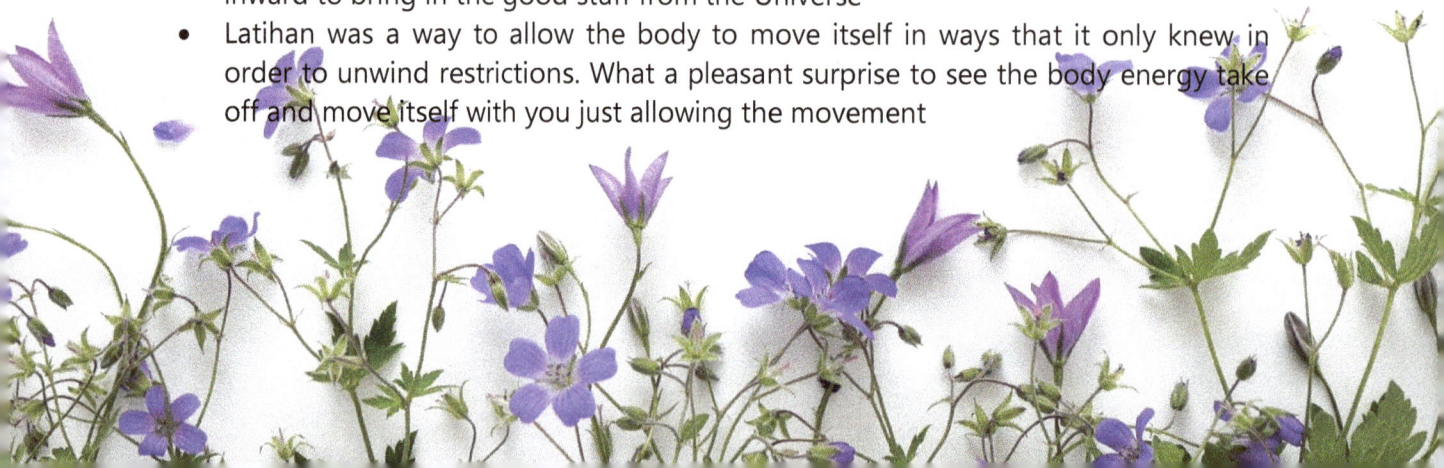

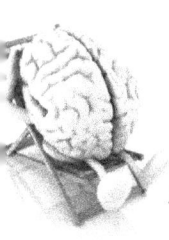

A few other helpful resources were:

- The Alchemical Hypnotherapy training where we learned how to access various depths of the subconscious, and to use a few different scenarios in order to find out underlying issues for unhappy emotional patterns or old wounds that kept resurfacing. This was super effective; so much so that by the end of it I pretty much felt like I'd had a happy childhood and felt grateful for it. For the finishing touches, in keeping with the 'web' of entanglements that Dr. Wonderly described that make change difficult, I developed something called:

- The 'Hall of Associations' - Using this method I was able to go down to the appropriate depth and open every door that had ever had a relationship to a particular pattern and clean out the debris in the room that was keeping that pattern tied to it. Emotional sides of earlier traumas never bothered me again, so mood swings, depression, and suicidal thoughts vanished.

- The Hanna Somatic Education training set the stage for a whole new way of creating change in the body. Improving communication between the brain and mechanoreceptors was a turning point in regaining the health that I'd lost in India. That system informed all my exercises from then on so they'd be seen as integrating input for the brain .

- Professional help. I'd worked with chiropractors and PT's during the 90's, enhancing my understanding of the rehab process and dealing with inflammation, plus they helped put my skeleton back where it belonged during the loose ligament phase.

- Satori through Grace – In a way, everything that came as a resource was a form of Grace. The several prolonged experiences of more sublime layers of consciousness provided a certain distance from identification with the injuries, as well as a space from which the mechanisms could be felt more clearly and supported from a place that was not injured. The active meditation period shifted into the capacity to sit still and silent for hours at a time, giving the nervous system a space of calm and support for reset.

- Diet was also a key resource. I learned that my system had not adapted well to being a vegetarian, and was malnourished as a result. The digestive disorders and intolerances that followed contributed to the lax ligaments, spasms, hypermobility of joints and vertebrae, and chronic inflammation. Reintroducing meat in my diet made a huge difference. It might not be for everyone, but for me, red meat was essential. It helped the foggy brain quite a bit in my case.

- Remaining active, respectful, and positive was very helpful. I'd discovered during the rehab of my back after India, that if I told my body it was doing great and getting stronger, it complied. I'd plant the thought that the pain would be pretty much gone in an hour, and it would be. I learned how to position myself to find the most neutral place while sitting, standing, or moving to minimize the strain, and I learned to respect the 'no-no's'.

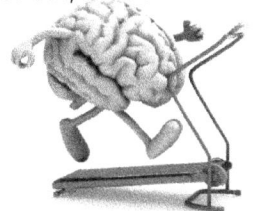

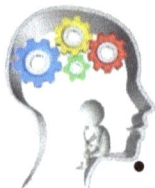

- Engaging my brain. I joined a performance band for three years in order to learn how to play the oboe, not only because I loved the sound (I was awful!), but also because I had to follow each note in time and remain focused. I played billiards when I could for the focus and eye-hand coordination, and played racquetball for the reflexes and speed needed to keep track of the ball, and the challenge to predict where the ball would land each time.

- Aerobic exercise. I danced, avoiding the movements that would agitate the neck or brain, and swam just a lap or two to smooth things out. And most recently, picked up bowling to wake up the areas that had fallen into auto-pilot, to learn something old in a new way, and for the focus. I sang and danced around the house every day, and stretched daily.

- Studying the brain. I was fortunate to learn about an osteopath who was offering classes, and though this was much later, taking Brain classes with Dr. Chikly was a real turning point in the healing process. I gave myself 6 months before the first class just to study the anatomy he'd laid out that would be covered in class to give my brain time to process and hold the information. That effort was a little painful and quite a struggle. I hadn't approached cognitive issues yet, but it's difficult to do when not thinking clearly is the problem.

- Studying the cranial system. Once again, friends recommended a training in the cranial sacral therapy modality, wherein many concussions have been known to have their symptoms improve. I spent three years in these classes.

- Studying rehabilitation. My mother's multiple infarct dementia wound up providing a lot of insight into how to rehabilitate the brain. During that decade or so (concurrent with my game-changer) I did constant research for her into supplements, exercises, nutritional support, along with consulting with a few doctors, nutritionists, acupuncturists, chiropractors, using energy medicine, physical and occupational therapists, biochemists, and naturopaths.

It was also during this time that I found out that it was possible to sense the brain and have an effect on the brainstem through the mouth. Her caregivers would often discuss things they'd tried with some of the other stroke patients, or some old family remedies they'd learned from their grandmothers back in their home country. The connection between the tongue and the brain stem came from that period of time, which was in itself a seed planted that gave a reminder of where to look to resolve my own injury ten years later. **Tip #5**: Inform yourself. Consider reading a book, listening to a webinar, or taking a class on how the body functions. It can transform anxiety into fascinating when faced with the 'unknown' parts of the process.

Even though it sounds like I had an advantage for recovery, I was also at a great disadvantage in that the injuries just kept coming even though I wasn't being a daredevil

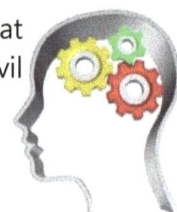

or putting myself in harm's way. I'm a firm believer in the saying that has the Universe being stacked in everyone's favor, and little things also kept happening that supported greater healing. When I overheard my chiropractor say to a patient, "Don't settle for less than 100%," that sentence set my mind up to expect my body to recover all the way. Total recovery became my goal, regardless of how it felt or how many injuries kept knocking on my door. I was determined to try whatever it took to get better and return to all the things I loved to do. **Tip #6**: Keep your eyes and ears open; life will always step in and offer hints.

At some point in the late 1990's my physical reserves were waning fast. The thing that may have contributed to things having a stronger effect and taking longer to heal might well have been the onset of menopause. Menopause changes everything because a major source of signaling and regulation has dropped in the number of worker bees available, and there's a downshift in metabolism. As mentioned earlier, the levels of tension in the muscles and connective tissue becomes unpredictable with hormonal changes, and neurological wobbles become a regular part of the week. The body is more vulnerable to inflammation because the drop in estrogen creates leaky gut which causes inflammation. All sorts of mysterious new aches and pains crop up.

The least favorite part of menopause for me was the hormonal insomnia. The sleep deprivation was so intense I'd go for days with 3-4 hours' sleep, then crash from exhaustion and get 6 hours. This went on for decades, so just know that while subsequent injuries are being described, they were trying to heal with half to one-third of the amount of sleep needed. The most famous by-product of menopause is that your memory goes down the tubes and brain farts are a regular occurrence. Vocabulary gaps are often filled in by 'thinga-majig', or 'hoochikoochie'.

A key ingredient that I learned and want to pass on, is that the symptoms of brain injury can be replicated to some degree by lack of proper nutrition, by lack of sleep, by hormonal imbalance, by neurotoxins, by your frame of mind, by EMF frequency disruption, by dehydration, and even lack of oxygen from vascular restrictions. Being able to understand and correct these contributing factors is the reason there can be so much improvement or reversal in brain-related dysfunctions. To a certain extent, continuing to improve these other areas of support gave my brain a chance to find resilience and plasticity again. **Tip #7**: Try not to expose your system to toxins or stressors that can be avoided, like fluoride, artificial sweeteners, MSG, pesticides and the like. It's easy enough to periodically check and see what your body's been exposed to using blood work, a saliva test, hair analysis, live blood cell test, or systemic scanners to see where the imbalances may be.

The second to the last straw
Keeping in mind that even though all of the previously listed resources going for me in

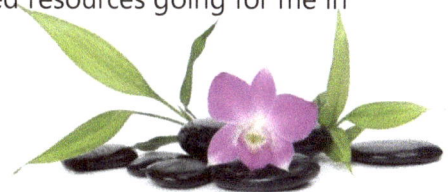

the 1990's, the year 2000 hits with a new wave of challenges that made earlier ones seem like boot camp for the real battle. Your body doesn't tell you that you're standing on a precipice. It's such a great strategist, it'll pull from here, there, and everywhere to keep you up and moving with adaptations. Looking back now, I can see that I had a couple more straws in my chest before the time ran out. It happened in less than a second. I hadn't been back long from the latest trip to India, and all was well that sunny afternoon.

I was proceeding into the intersection on a green light when a pickup truck slammed into my driver's side door. There was a sideways whiplash with my head banging against the window of that door, which was badly damaged in the crash. I managed to force the door open to check in with the driver of the truck. The driver in the blue pickup stopped for a moment on the other side of the street, but took off when I got out of the car. My attention shifted to my body to see how it was doing, as the shock was wearing off and I wanted to see how to minimize the effects of the impact. There wasn't a lot of immediate pain. I remembered some of my queries while at the physical therapy clinics about the forces going through the car and landing in the bodies of the passengers, and decided to immediately begin shaking my body to discharge those forces.

A few bystanders came over and the police arrived. It's funny how you hear different interpretations of the same event, and some even remembered the color of the truck differently. The officer pretty much told me 'fat chance' of getting anything from the driver, since there were too many of these types of accidents each month to keep up with them, he said. As it turned out the plates didn't belong to the truck anyway. I went home and stretched, took a bath in Epsom salts and waited to see how things materialized in my body. I went to work the next day which was with an orthopedic chiropractor who gave me a few adjustments and recommended taking ibuprofen, which would be the first time for me. Since I rarely took anything for pain, they worked right away. In three weeks practically all of the symptoms had waned and life was back to normal. The next time things went a little differently, and I'll always believe it was because I was in a hurry and didn't take time to shake the forces out of my system.

Resources face emptying reserves

Once my reserves and capacity to compensate and bounce back had been used up, my system became a magnet for mishaps. My threshold for pain was greatly reduced while the sensitivity had exponentially increased. It was as if my system was broadcasting on that frequency and just kept replaying the same song. The series of 'hits' went like this for the next 25 years, but I'll just list the top ten and what worked the best in each case.

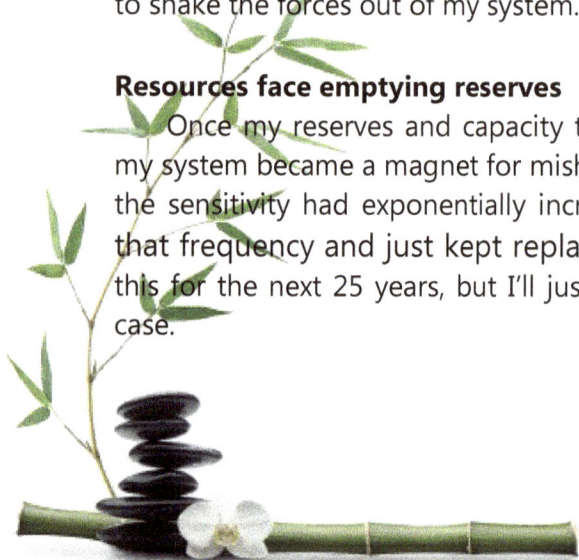

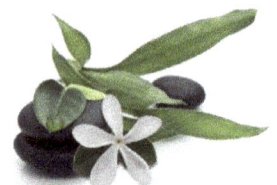

1. **Sprained right ankle**
   I began to play racquetball again and found a tennis partner to keep the heart rate up. I rolled my ankle and heard a pop
   Symptoms: Pain, swelling, can't walk without limping
   Treatment: Ice, elevation, ace bandage, DMSO, Traumeel (homeopathic anti-inflammatory), and proteolytic enzymes (for swelling and adhesions)
   What really helped the most: Doing all of it daily

2. **Time to heal:** 3 weeks
   Rear-end whiplash – Coup/Contra coup
   Sitting at a stop sign someone rear-ended me. I was on my way to the vet with my cat in the car that was freaking out, so I didn't do my little shaking to get the forces out of my system
   Symptoms: Pain and inflammation down the right side to the sacrum, increased sensitivity on the right side of the face, tongue, jammed temporal bone, trigger points in the neck, shoulder and back; disc protrusions onto thecal sac of cord at C4 & 5; cervical vertebrae lost their curve;
   Treatment: Chi Kung, Chiropractic using (rapid thrust), massage, micro-neural current, ultrasound
   What helped the most: Trigger point work, Paul St. John's NeuroMuscular therapy working the anterior cervical muscles, Chi Kung with modified movements emphasizing each articulation of the spine in gentle, specific sequences, and micro-neural current
   Side–effects: Strain and irritation to denticulate ligaments and paraspinals using rapid thrust method in chiropractic
   Time to heal: One year

3. **Front end whiplash – Coup/Contra coup**
   An elder who couldn't see or hear well leaves his stop sign while I'm exiting the freeway and I swerved, but still crash into his passenger door. Head hits the steering wheel, and my right knee hits the dash
   Symptoms: Face and head pain, some pain in the right knee, numbness and tingling in left hand and fingers, neck and 'brain' pain which the nurse said wasn't possible; very heavy, difficult to lift arms and legs, thoracic outlet
   Treatment: Lymph drainage, Chiropractic with activator and drop table, ice, Traumeel and other natural topical anti-inflammatories, a neurologist visit who recommended acupuncture and a shoulder brace for thoracic outlet symptoms; other chiropractor for head pain; osteopathy; knee brace; began working on cervical curve with visualization and lying on a rolled up towel
   What helped the most: Lymph drainage enabled arms to lift easily again; activator served the heaviness in legs; and topical anti-inflammatories; osteopathy helped the numbness and face/head pain; old neck stiffness from childhood falls resolved

with activator and osteopathy

Side-effects: Drop-table technique aggravated facial bones and increased pain; chiropractic attempts to decompress cranial bones made head pain worse; moved to a place without so many stairs to nurse the knee

Time to heal: concurrent with the last injury so an additional six months

4. **Backwards Fall – Concussion – Sudden Deceleration**

In this case someone had hosed down the redwood deck so it was slippery. While going to light candles, I hit the beam on the arbor with my forehead, but couldn't catch my balance on the wet deck so fell hard like on ice.

Symptoms: shock, pain all over the spine and sacrum; saw stars, inability and fear to move

Treatment: Osteopathy, Somatics, Chi kung, proteolytic enzymes, ibuprofen and exercise (aerobic), Chiropractic with myofascial and cranial focus

What helped the most: They all helped

Time to heal: Hard to tell; it was an uncomfortable time

5. **Pass Out and Fall – Sudden Deceleration (This one's the last straw!)**

I was playing tennis and something went funny in my chest that absorbed my brain; everything was getting fuzzy and going white so I went to sit down and put my head between my knees. Drank some water and felt better but when I stood up the spell was coming on again so I grabbed the chain link fence and later opened my eyes with people saying, "She's coming to!" My first reaction was to yell and grab the back of my head.

Symptoms: Major pain in my head and spine, initially, then loss of balance, aphasia, dyslexia, stuttering, stammering, sensitivity to light and sound on the right side, trigeminal neuralgia, hemiplegic migraines on the right, black outs or blank outs, big-time confusion about time and space, PTSD, trembling with exercise, fatigue from talking, using the computer for too long tightened my throat and burned the eyes, ADHD, vasovagal episodes (dizzy spells with intense left side weakness, numbness, pain, spasm, sweat), difficulty hearing in restaurants or crowded places, no dreams – just blank. Since much of the force went anterior with the posterior impact, my earlier injury with the slug to the throat and possibly tonsillectomy came into play and made for a very difficult period to use my voice without exhaustion; inflammation & irritation of 6 cranial nerves

Treatment: CT scan, Osteopathic, ibuprofen, hypericum (homeopathic for nerve pain), Neuroheel, Chiropractic neurology using eye exercises and supplements, a metronome and other methods, sacred geometry, light therapy, low-frequency neurofeedback, EMDR, brain exercises, hemi-sync brain wave frequencies, acupuncture, colorpuncture, red meat (advised by neurologist), Rolfing, Zero Balancing, Hawthorne berry extract, adaptogens

What helped the most: Light therapy (using the color my brain preferred which

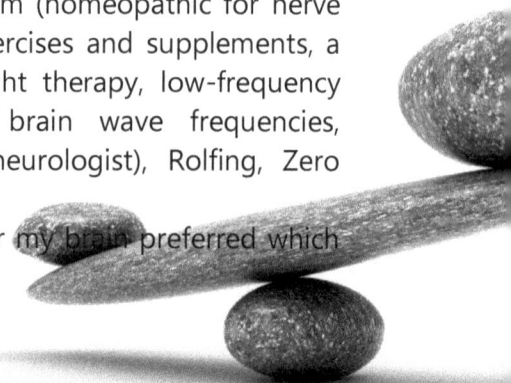

was purple), osteopathy – particularly in the mouth and freeing the neck, Rolfing under the tongue, protecting the ears and eyes from light and sound; being in quiet Nature – like the desert or redwoods, meditation, gentle, moderate exercise, work on the brain and particularly the cerebellum, sacral hold and down-regulation of the nervous system with Cranial Sacral, Neurofeedback, and a brainwave CD that generated more Delta waves and enhanced sleep, red meat, sacred geometry, especially on airplanes, in hotel rooms, and near electronic devices; time

Time it took to heal: Five to 6 years – 85% healed with retrigger upon lack of sleep or big stress, which are related - or non-expert touch of my neck

6. **Forehead Coup/Contra coup**

For some reason, a glass and metal shower door became unhinged just as I was approaching it and fell onto my forehead. This was not long after the game-changer

Symptoms: Just a mass of spasm, inflammation, and pain

Treatment: Massage, Pap-imi device (high frequency treatment using millivolts), polychromatic light box

What helped me most: polychromatic light box

Side-effects: but the red frequency from that light box gave me a migraine – my back felt great though

Time it took to heal: The light box erased spasms and back pain in an hour, but it set back the progress of the game-changer

7. **Top of the Head Impacts**

Maybe by this time Murphy's Maxim is having a field day, because stuff started falling off of shelves onto the top of my head - like a picture frame, or a piece of wood in the shed

Symptoms: These were very difficult in a different way. Cervical pain and compression, pain in cranial sutures, cranial bone compression, throat tension, replication of whiplash symptoms, trigger points and their referred pain lit up in upper right quadrant and head, sciatica, and engagement of back muscles all down the right side

Treatment: Osteopathic work, Somatic exercises, Contemplation, Chi kung, aerobic exercise, plus did my own trigger points and manual therapy

What helped the most: Everything helped

Side-effects: I discovered a spot on the right side of the neck near C4 that got very tight, but could trigger head trauma pain with trigger points if pressed (perhaps near that bulging disc?); and the area in the thoracic outlet space above the left clavicle that triggered the vasovagal episode a few times

Time it took to heal: A few months

Sidebar: Somewhere in this time frame my dreams returned but as matter-of-fact representations of the day – nothing symbolic or prophetic

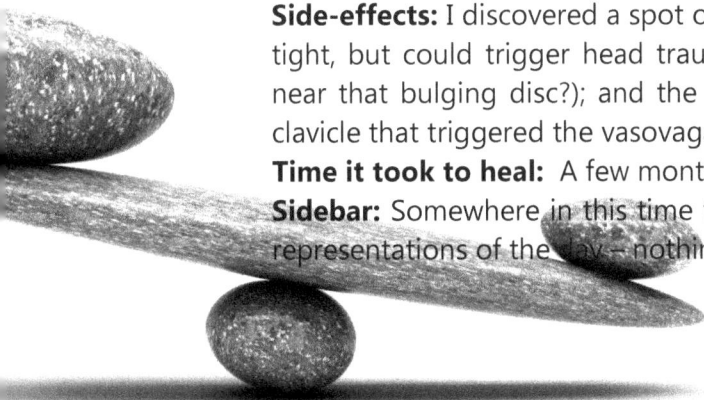

8. **Front End Crash** This one was my fault. We were cruising along in traffic and I turned my attention for a fraction of a second to pick up a snack to eat and when I turned back the airbag was in my face. The seat belt forced a three-dimensional metal necklace into my sternum and the airbag smashed my sunglasses into my nose, then off my face

Symptoms: Intense, immediate chest pain, disorientation, shock, face pain, difficulty sleeping because my ribs hurt so much to lie on them, numbness and tingling down left arm and hand; something not right with vasculature above the heart and the liver was upset on the left lobe; esophagus effected and began often choking on food and drink

Treatment: Everything in mishap #7

What helped the most: Meditation, contemplation, manual therapy, topical anti-inflammatories

Time to heal: A few more months

Side bar: By this time I was completing a training in Biodynamic Cranial Sacral Therapy and was able to receive treatment the same day. It was amazing to feel that the fluids and fascia had taken on a velcro-like quality and were truly stuck together, just like the textbooks say it does. There was quite the burning sensation as the fluids tried to permeate the trauma

9. **Cranial Base Impact #1 with Falling Object**

Murphy still had it in for me when I bent over in the closet to retrieve a pair of summer shoes from the bottom of it and the vacuum cleaner came loose from its hook and tagged me in the back of the head on the right side.

Symptoms: Head and neck pain, and a line of irritation and inflammation going all the way down the left side capturing the path of the bladder and gall bladder meridians down the back and side of the leg to the toes; dura and cord contraction was so powerful that I lost an inch and a half of height, spatial disorientation, loss of balance

Treatment: Osteopathy, activator chiropractic, stretching, contemplation and meditation, manual therapy on myself, Somatic movements, enzymes

What worked best this time: By now I'm in Brain classes which was quite helpful, so used all of the above, but only one or two sessions from outside practitioners

Time to heal: A few weeks

Side bar: My dreams are becoming symbolic again, although the brain gets overly stimulated and wakes me up in the middle every time REM sleep shows up

10. **Cranial Base Impact #2 with Falling Object**

This would have worked way better if I hadn't just been slammed on the other side. In this case a clay flower pot full of dirt fell off a shelf onto the back of my head while I was bent over getting some dirt out of a sack.

Symptoms: This one seemed to go back and recreate every other head injury I'd ever had. I was beginning to feel really sorry for my poor neck. Just go back through the list and add every type of pain, inflammation, and spasm I'd ever had in the past and bring it forward, minus the hemiplegic migraines and trigeminal neuralgia. The trigeminal nerve was irritated and the referred pain in the head and suture pain was off the charts.

Treatment: A couple of osteopathic treatments, an activator session for my neck and sacrum; serrapeptase, ice, Traumeel, my own manual therapy, contemplation, Chi kung, plus herbal support, systemic enzymes, brain work in class, continued aerobic exercise, hyperbaric oxygen chamber, trigger points

What helped the most: Probably at this point just being very diligent in working with it every day and every night, and releasing the main forces of the trauma and compression along the skull and spine with practitioners who by now knew my body very well; also, working directly on releasing cellular trauma in the brain class as well as focusing on specific nuclei, particularly the cerebellum and geniculate bodies, was a remarkable help

Time to heal: A few months

Side-effects: I'd been taking systemic (proteolytic) enzymes for a few years to help with inflammation and scar tissue, but I'd noticed that blood vessels in my hands were popping and bruising in a painful way a few times a week.

Side bar: When I asked the teacher of the osteopathic training about the blood vessels bursting, he mentioned that the amount of lipase might be too much in those enzymes. I cut back on enzymes with high amounts of lipase and the issue went away. I used serrapeptase (one of the ingredients) by itself after that, which was the best for nerve pain in my system.

As trauma situations accumulated in the middle age years, the earlier surgeries, falls, and injuries began to show themselves. The pain patterns that my nervous system had previously subdued and limiting fascial were showing up again. The injuries and surgeries in the throat, nasal cavity, and belly were making noise on a regular basis during the latter head traumas, but could also often be instrumental in releasing an entire web of tension. **Tip #8:** See if you can notice which areas are repeating strain patterns and connect that area in a movement sequence or in a stretch with your center of gravity and legs. Differentiate types of pain if you can, because they respond differently to the type of intervention; i.e. nerve pain, inflammation, spasming muscles, referred pain, pain from compression, etc.

Subcutaneous nerve pain responds well to skin rolling, vessel wall pain likes stretching of the artery, suture pain responds to ice and anti-inflammatories, referred pain needs trigger point work, and so on. At this point I'd already taken a few osteopathic classes, visceral classes, and brain classes, an osteopathic training, not only because I was

Right anterior cerebral artery

Anterior communicating artery

Right internal carotid artery

Left middle cerebral artery

Right posterior communicating artery

Right posterior cerebral artery

Arterial circle

Basilar artery

Spinal cord

Left vertebral artery

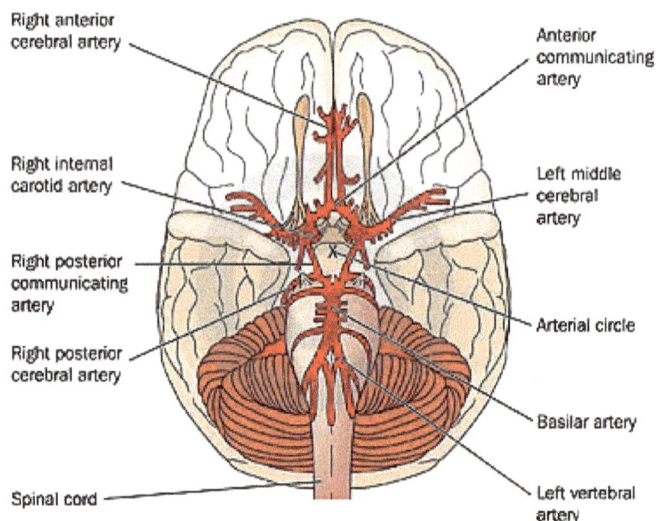

concerned about my well-being going forward, but also because I was excited about that body of work. I was getting treated in classes 4 to 6 times a year, all day for a few days in a row. In some cases, like with the brain and classes focusing on bones and connective tissue (moreso than muscles, which seemed more reflexive than causative) I felt better than ever, so was motivated to keep learning and exploring.

Working a few days on the cerebellum in the brain class got rid of tinnitus I'd had for decades from being in a rock band in the 70's and 80's, and turned the tide toward brain balance in a major way. Quite a bit of force from the whiplashes and impacts to the back of the head landed in my blood vessels, so the vascular class was one of the most soothing experiences of them all. Not only that, the class enhanced the flow of oxygen into the brain, including the Circle of Willis, which intersects with several other arteries at the base of the brain, an area often indicated in brain trauma. Studying different modalities revealed their influence in the global web. I also learned that less is probably more in the acute phase or exacerbation of an injury, since the system can become easily overloaded and create pain just from the level of stimulation it was receiving in a short amount of time. **Tip #9**: Consider developing a meditation practice, as there was no treatment or medication or supplement that could accomplish the same calm in the brain.

There was another reason for taking all those classes related to rebalancing the system. It was partly because all those treatments would have been expensive, and many of those practitioners didn't bill insurance. I figured I'd get more out of it in the long run if I understood more about the principles and mechanisms that made the techniques effective, then I could not only use them to help my clients, but I could also use them on myself when possible (which was every day). Trying to get my brain on board again to study and absorb new information was like dragging a log uphill in the rain every single day of each class. It was very stressful in an indescribable sort of way as well as being exhausting since my brain was still out of shape cognitively and struggling at every turn.

Recovery in that sense was similar to rehabilitating my back after the disc injury and finding out what it could tolerate and what it couldn't do without exacerbation. It took a few years, but much of that was due to over-use setbacks and the wrong diet. In other words, much of what worked for rehabilitating my brain was understood through trial and error, through educated guessing, and through following the research as it emerged in recent years. There are layers to an injury. Once the damage recedes and the pain subsides, there's a period of getting strong, integrated, and functioning normally again. After settling the pain and agitation in the brain and nervous system, the spatial and balance issues begin to reset, but need specific conscious movements to do so. Cognitive reeducation is a different layer and requires a separate and different form of exercises.

I guess part of what lasted the longest as a symptom is a type of fatigue through sensory overload. I just didn't let myself or my brain rest enough and fatigued my eyes and ears over and over again. I've continued to wear sunglasses in all but dark, cloudy or evening skies, and in fluorescent lighting. This is one thing that's remained sensitive for forty years. My ears recovered much more easily. It's like the need to find the balance between challenging the brain so it can retain plasticity, and resting it so it can restore and cleanse itself. I still take many hours each day to spend quietly and alone, with limited stimulation in the evening. I rarely go out to socialize since socializing meant talking, and talking was fatiguing.

When not in an acute phase and the symptoms were abating, I did continue to see my osteopath a couple of times a year for preventive measure. Some areas on the backside of the body just can't easily be reached and would require someone else to facilitate release in those areas; not only that, their skill level and knowledge base will be beyond what your own hands on your body could accomplish. Another key incentive for continuing treatment was that the earlier punch in my jaw created a great deal of shuffling in my lower teeth. They were all over the place with some teeth heading anterior and some heading posterior. Using Invisalign to correct the position of the teeth put an enormous amount of pressure on the skull, and created setbacks a few times.

It continued to be a pleasant surprise that meditation still proved to be such a great resource to strengthen and reset the system. Even if a virus was coming on, a meditative contemplation of where the virus was trying to enter could 9 times out of 10 rebalance that area and ward off the virus. The notion that there was a seamless continuity physiologically, neurologically, energetically, emotionally, and structurally with different layers of consciousness was ever intriguing. The fact that the subtler layers of consciousness were interacting with regulatory systems in a way that could have a profound influence on health was deeply motivating. It kept me in classes, in spiritual practices, and in front of spiritual teachers for decades.

That doesn't mean that others can't benefit greatly from the methods used without studying the methods, or without embarking on a spiritual journey, because most healing methods have at their base a spiritual component. I happen to be a curious person anyway, and the years of lying awake unable to sleep either due to hormonal changes or pain lent themselves to inquiry and contemplation into the sources of the pain and how to connect those areas to health again. I found it fascinating. I'll list what worked for me and maybe from there you can get some ideas of what to try for your own situation.

Self-treating options

Sensations are heightened during any form of injury. The Somatics work in neuromuscular reeducation had at its foundation the intention to give the brain information through its sensory apparatus. There is always the possibility of helping to guide the brain back into feeding forward its more normal baseline for muscles and connective tissue by using these sensations. Both the chiropractor that I'd worked for as well Tom Hanna had treated ankle injuries manually immediately after it happened to reduce scarring and encourage normalcy. Initially skeptical about using direct methods in an acute phase of an injury, I recently turned my left ankle again and decided to try it.

I waited a beat to get a sense of how serious it was, but at this point both ankles have such stretched out ligaments that I could practically walk on them with the soles of my feet facing each other. That being said, the searing, burning pain was getting started and I immediately introduced a stabilizing hold at the subtalar joint, then just beneath the malleoli (ankle bones) and avoided soft tissue. The bones are responsible for a great deal of the immune response right after an injury so I had the sense that it would be a better place to start. Releasing forces from bone can also help to reset the soft tissue around it.

As the pain was decreasing rather than increasing, I added the pandiculation method that Hanna Somatics made famous. Perhaps similar in principle to muscle energy, pandiculation encompasses a wider range of motion as a way of sending input to the brain about the length of the tissue and position of the joint. Self-sensing movement awareness exercises that are gentle and therefore non-threatening can intervene before the tissue field sets up in a pattern of guarding or compensation that winds up being counter-productive. I've found it to be very effective in decreasing pain in tight, sore muscles, but hadn't tried in this context yet where more ligaments than muscles were involved. In any case, it immediately reset the joint to the point where I forgot that I tweaked it. It's different for the brain in an acute phase for many reasons. One obvious reason is that you can't directly put your hands on it, and it's figuratively a muscle, but not literally.

There are still ways to be in touch with the brain to guide it towards restoration of balance and normal functioning. One way is to release the forces that may have sheared

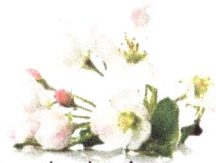

up in the surrounding membranes that might be rotating, compressing, or tilting the brain. Another way to reduce the consequences of a recent head injury is to facilitate proper motion of the cranial bones and their reciprocal motion, in cases where it's a closed head injury and there's no fractured skull or hematomas. Finding ways to discharge the shock and agitation in the cells can be very helpful. Treating fluid systems, meditating, and working with the breath can serve this purpose.

Each client who I've worked with through the years who's been interested in self-treating has been able to discern their own fluid and organ motion with guidance. There are also more indirect ways to release pressure from the skull and brain by opening up the fascial planes that run from one end of the body to the other, as well as using muscular groups that connect to the neck and head. This is pretty easy to do through gentle movements that access the spine by using the extremities. Inclusive, conscious movement also serves to encourage integration of the system rather than allowing the injury to determine the course of events throughout the tissue field. Suggested movements come a little later in the text.

Because the osteopath who worked with most of my injuries over 25 years started with the bones in the feet and balanced the skeleton all the way up including the ribs before adjusting or mobilizing cranial bones and membranes, I could feel the way my body responded to this approached compared to those who went straight for the skull. She also worked on the anterior cervicals and inside the mouth which releases an enormous amount of pressure from the head. I learned from those methods that were the most relieving in the acute phases, what I needed to do to produce the same relief, although I would see her first right after the injury, then move into self-treating. It was definitely trial and error, as I made some boo-boos along the way and caused pain. Whenever possible, I worked inside my own mouth using little finger cots from the drug store to soften the masseter and pterygoids, to clear tensions under the tongue, balance the hard palate, and release the vomer. Understanding the connections of the anterior cervical fascia to the hyoid and cricoid was incredibly helpful to the release and balance, along with connections down the arm that could tighten the upper traps that are innervated by the spinal accessory cranial nerve (which could easily become impacted in a fall).

The traps originate at the nuchal line(s) on the occiput which could potential pull on the skull whenever the arms are being used. If the anatomical terms are unfamiliar, don't hesitate to ask your practitioner to show you where they are and the best ways to access them on yourself. You can practice one method or one area at a time until you feel comfortable and confident that you have the knack. Toward the latter few injuries I had a pretty good sense of how head injuries circulated in my system, and had tried so many things It was fairly clear (until these new revelations) what to use to help them release. By

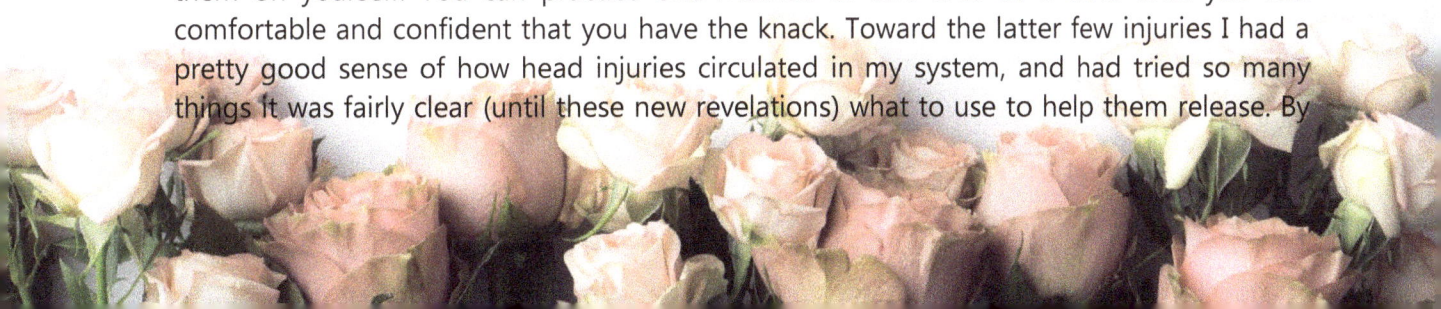

then I usually only went to one osteopathic and one chiropractic session and orchestrated the rest of the rehab myself. Most things are accessible through movement, breath, and meditation, but it certainly helps to have a professional kick-start the process first.

I also learned to distinguish different types of pain and knew to treat certain types with ice and systemic enzymes or serrapeptase, or extinguishing trigger points even before going to the osteopath. You can Google 'trigger point map' to find out if your pain is referring according to one of those patterns, then apply gentle, repeated pressure on it until it gradually recedes. Icing the point could also help it to desensitize. It's worth every moment of effort it takes to stay alert during painful episodes in order to learn from them and how your body responds so that self-treating can begin to flourish. Pain and inflammation become less scary when you have a sense of why they're there and understand how to get rid of them.

At its finest, the Biodynamic model attunes the system to its inherent healing forces ever present in the fluids that transport waste, nourishment, endogenous analgesics, immune support, and energy. It can also align the bony structures to remove restrictions, and can mobilize those inherent forces optimally to facilitate the system's self-regulatory capacities. Once a relationship is established between you and your body, it isn't difficult to enhance your own fluids using subtle touch. I've settled my nervous system many a night by holding my sacrum and base of the skull, waiting for the CSF rhythm to gain more potency. In my earlier books, "Somatic Intelligence" volumes 4 and 5, I go into great detail about how to establish a deeper relationship of listening and responding to your body, and how to develop sensitivity to the sensations it produces.

Using contemplation as a form of treatment

Contemplation is very similar to meditation, in that the practitioner is really being a witness to the goings-on in the system while holding space and observing how it responds to a stimulus that makes it aware of itself. They say that an object changes when the observer is present, and that certainly seems to be true, as if some subtle form of intelligence is 'listening' to and responding to your every touch and intent, using its own programing to orient itself to restoration, but also following the promptings of the practitioner's repository of knowledge. A Chi Kung instructor once said, "Energy goes where attention goes." From this perspective, contemplating your system is also sending energy to the areas that need it. Many times the area will begin to soften and let go as soon as your attention reaches it. As you can imagine, it's rewarding to discover where pain comes from in any given situation.

I tried to learn what changed the sensation and which system was being affected in the varying types of pain. In some cases the pain was in the sutures of the skull, at times in the cranial nerves, and often in the areas the cranial nerves served. Frequently after a whiplash or superior to inferior injury, trigger points lit up like a Christmas tree and referred pain up and down the body in their respective patterns. The most common were in the sternocleidomastoids that referred to the top of the head, and the ones all around the shoulder blades. After the nervous system was settled, the shock discharged, and the trigger points resolved, there wasn't much pain left.

Once it was de-mystified the pain could be resolved in a few weeks, including the wide-spread contraction patterns up and down one side of the body, depending upon which side of the brain took the hit. Although muscle tension and contractions were also present, it was not the type of pain that a massage could influence for long since the contractions were stimulated by hyper-arousal of various brain cells. Working with the sensory-motor cortex at the top of the head and following the descending fibers down through the corona radiate across to the midbrain reliably softens the paraspinals, as does releasing the jaws, but adding movement that feeds back to the brain is necessary for those releases to sustain. Aerobic exercise, Feldenkrais movement, or Chi kung each help in different ways.

Yoga can be too intense for head trauma initially, as so many of the postures twist the spine and have the head down below the knees adding a great deal of pressure to the brain. Once the initial pain is gone and the after-contractions have subsided it can be helpful, but even then it's usually best to start slow and take it easy, not trying to keep up with a class, but doing an inner yoga, if you will, tracking and releasing inner tensions and restrictions with awareness. After the blows to the top of the head it felt like my meridians hurt, particularly the bladder, gall bladder, and Governing vessel. Chi kung and Shiatsu are most helpful for these kinds of energetic imbalances that cause pain. There's more detail about working with meridians later in the text.

Treating these long meridians reliably helped restore motion of the cranial bones and erector spinae or paraspinal muscles. Although I could also have an effect on these unilateral contractions by discharging the 'buzz' in the brain or certain nerve plexus like the brachial plexus, and the parasympathetic plexus at the sacrum, it was equally effective to palm the eyes, to hold the brain stem, or to relax my jaws. Besides those key areas, focusing on the fibers at the end of the spinal cord (cauda equine and filum terminale) until they soften and lengthen does wonders for the dural tension at the opposite end. These would usually be my 'go tos' in the middle of the night when I'd reliably awaken at 4 o'clock in the morning, and I'd be able to go back to sleep afterwards.

The more challenging aspects of head trauma were the post-concussive symptoms that come later. For one thing, you weren't sure what they were going to be. I could tell when I would stumble around off balance, or the dyslexia would show up in phone numbers, math would suddenly draw a blank, the halted speech would come, or those dreaded blank outs would sneak in. For those, the brain nutrition, aerobic exercise, and eye-hand coordination activities that required presence and focus would usually bring things back to normal. Lack of sleep could bring back balance and spatial issues, or even halted speech if sleep-deprived for days in a row, so rest and natural sleep aids are always helpful.

Coming into present day, after a lifetime of at least 50 traumatic incidents, most of which involved impacts to the head, the only remaining symptoms are brain fatigue with over-use of the computer, which causes eye strain and tightening of my throat, as does having lengthy conversations. My right knee has been fine with stairs for the last ten or so years, but needs attention from time to time. Sleep is still challenging because I have to lie on my head and neck. My right ankle is still weaker, but responds well to reeducation. Most nights for the last couple of years I get 6 to 8 hours with some REM sleep, but that's heavenly compared to the 2 to 4 hours it was for two decades.

Extra-curricular activities include walking, occasional jogging or calisthenics, dancing, swimming, basketball, racquetball, gardening, and now bowling. Maybe because it was a new activity, and partly because the weight of the ball pulled right up to the neck and head, rest was needed initially between games, a light ball worked best, and at times I'd stretch and shake it out in between frames. It's helpful to recognize the difference between regular fatigue and brain fatigue. For me it was best not to bowl when either type is present. With brain fatigue, other symptoms might begin to show up like slowed speech, loss of balance, brain fog, reduced vocabulary, tension at the back of the throat, sounds become irritating, and others, depending upon how it may have evolved in your individual system.

One of my brain injury clients takes naps in the afternoon, wears sunglasses indoors and keeps artificial lights low in the evening. I could barely speak initially after bowling and if I played three rather than two games, there was hell to pay the next day. After 8 weeks three games was fine as was the socializing part of the game. A type of global tension also accompanies brain fatigue; the whole body tightens - but runs along familiar patterns that can be undone. Many functional neurologists will recommend going slowly into exercise and to stop before reaching that point, and that's definitely a good idea if you recognize the signs. A little challenge is good to stretch the envelope from time to time, but the brain is perhaps a more delicate rehabilitation process than a shoulder injury.

Initially with bowling there was a motivation to get a little more exercise, to see if I could be more consistent by developing better form, and to add an activity that required mental focus. Then I felt the countless mini-stresses and strains, stiffnesses and awkwardness toward moving in a new way. Watching my brain struggle to set aside old movement patterns and attend to a new, very specific possibility was a most fascinating learning process in neurological awakening and integration. **Tip #10:** Adding something new can be supremely awakening for your brain and entire body, and reveal underused or undiscovered restricted areas.

Bowling became like deconstructing the entire sequence of walking and throwing a ball and rebuilding it fiber by fiber, joint by joint, cell by cell - not to become a pro, but to see how much this system could reorganize itself in a brand new way and forget its concussions, age, and predispositions. It was also an inquiry into the bridging between the mechanics of consciousness in the body and the consciousness that transcends the body and the brain. It was a test to see if intention and inherent plasticity can supersede the inherent psychological and neurological tendency to follow the path of least resistance. The global, integrating movements that followed becoming aware of the sticky places that bowling made more obvious were invaluable. Now there's no pain, only stiffness and contractions that arise from an over-stimulated or fatigued brain.

Three categories of contemplation:
1. The first category involves sitting quietly and sensing past the areas of tension into an inner silent zone. By dropping into that still, open space behind the tension, the body would relax as if there was a string binding it that suddenly let go. (Similar to focusing on the sky instead of the houses, telephone poles, billboards, etc.)
2. Another way the contemplation could happen would be sensing each area that had felt like bump in an otherwise smooth landscape. By putting awareness on both the bump and the smooth, empty adjacent terrain at the same time, the bump would let go into the empty surround. (Like ice dissolving in water.)
3. The third way includes sensing a bump in relationship to another bump in the landscape, which could be anywhere in the terrain. I'd search for a similar sensation with the premise that if the sensations were similar, they were both experiencing a similar type of strain that may have come as they were engaged at the same time. (Like two objects tangled into one another sitting too high in a drawer preventing the drawer from being able to open)

A fourth way that revealed itself in the process of contemplating in the other three methods was seeing that some tension patterns were tied to thought, particularly in the spine and joints. Often when the other bumps began to smooth out there would be a central or core tension that felt connected to the corpus callosum, or something right in the center of the brain that contracts when the brow is furrowed while thinking about

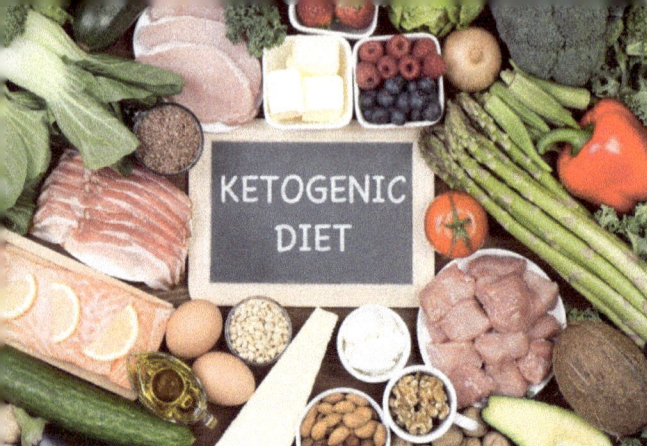

something. That furrowed brow can settle in to an unconscious ongoing subtle contraction during a busy period when there might be a lot on your mind. Thinking literally pulls the two hemispheres of the brain toward each other as the information passes between them, creating a little tightening of the dura that works its way all the way down the spinal cord.

Using these three zones of contemplating restrictions or contractions in my system opened and lengthened my spine to the extent that the inch and a half lost after the ten more recent, major hits was almost all regained. What will it take to maintain consciousness not only of the body, but in the body? It takes regular practice. Repetitive, gentle, slow, conscious movement that engages all of the joints simultaneously, or still, meditative contemplation of the sensation of tension patterns creates such a fluid integration of the system that it literally feels like you're floating while you walk, like you're opposing gravity.

Nutrition possibilities for the brain

Nutrition can make or break the difference in the recovery of any number of conditions including brain injuries. I remember so clearly the craving that got set up in my brain after the stimulation of the neurofeedback treatments. Each time my system wanted water and something sweet immediately after, making me think that glucose, the brain's energy source, and hydration were pretty significant for the brain returning to normal functioning. Of course, it should be a healthier source of glucose than the ones I chose during that craving, but the point was taken. Instead of store-bought chocolate, I began making my own organic dark chocolate bars with cocoa butter, cocoa powder, açai powder, nuts, honey, dried fruit, cardamom, cinnamon, and a little peppermint or orange oil. As a potent source of magnesium and antioxidants, dark chocolate is getting a lot of good press lately.

There is a little controversy out there over which form of glucose to take in, and most denounce processed sugar and especially artificial sweeteners, which can be quite toxic for the brain. Many current scientists, doctors, and nutritionists are suggesting the ketogenic diet that includes quite a bit of protein and fat burning as a source of fuel. In support of this position, there are some anecdotal reports of coconut oil reversing signs of Alzheimer's and you likely can't go wrong with quality fish oil. Some may recommend whole grains due to the B vitamins and fiber, whereas others discourage the inclusion of grains due to the gluten content that could contribute to inflammation. Sweet potatoes and yams have a host of benefits and could be a healthy source of carbs, and some recommend beans that are soaked first. At the end of the day, it's best to take everything under advisement and check in with what your system seems the respond the best to. **Tip #11:** Feed your brain.

I began including brain foods in my diet on a regular basis whether I had post-concussion symptoms or not. While in the midst of them, ginger works wonders for suture pain headaches as well as for nausea coming with a head injury. Walnuts and blueberries were one of my favorites, along with essential fatty acids, green powders, anti-oxidants, B, C, and E vitamins, D3, tumeric, gotu kola, tulsi, and Brahmi. D- ribose, NAC (N-Acetyl Cysteine to boost glutathione levels), L Carnitine, PQQ, and CoQ10 found their way to my regime for heart and mitochondria support, along with various detox and blood purifying assistance like dandelion root, cat's claw, Pau d'Arco, and red clover blossoms.

I use a variety of healthy fat oils, but gravitate towards black seed oil, olive oil, sacha inchi oil, sesame oil and coconut oil. Ashwaghanda, Dead Sea Salt baths, astragalus, trace minerals, magnesium and probiotics supported my stress levels along with trusty high quality vitamin C and vitamin E with tocotrienols. Mind you, some of these things (and a few others I didn't mention) I take once or twice a month, some once or twice a week, and some every few weeks, but the raw, organic veggie juice with anti-oxidant or supergreen powders and liquid trace minerals are usually every day. I try to follow what my body is asking for or open to rather than following a preset formula. Too many herbs or herbal teas tended to irritate my kidneys, but I didn't notice the same thing with basic (food sourced) vitamins and mineral supplements. I'm working on increasing water intake. **Tip#12**: Listen to your body.

BDNF (brain-derived neurotrophic factor) is all the rage now for the support of brain function, in that it helps glucose and lipid metabolism. Researchers at the National Institute of Health report that, *"BDNF is an excellent example of a signaling molecule that is intimately related to both energy metabolism and synaptic plasticity; it can engage in metabolic activity.... and is most abundant in areas of the brain associated with cognitive and metabolic function, namely the hippocampus and hypothalamus."* (Dr. Fernando Gomez-Pinilla, *"Brain foods: the effects of nutrients on brain function"*, The National Review of Neuroscience", July 2008) The simplest way to increase BDNF levels is to exercise, to employ intermittent fasting if it suits your blood sugar levels, and to consume egg yolks if you can.

Although excess could create problems, grass fed red meat minus antibiotics and

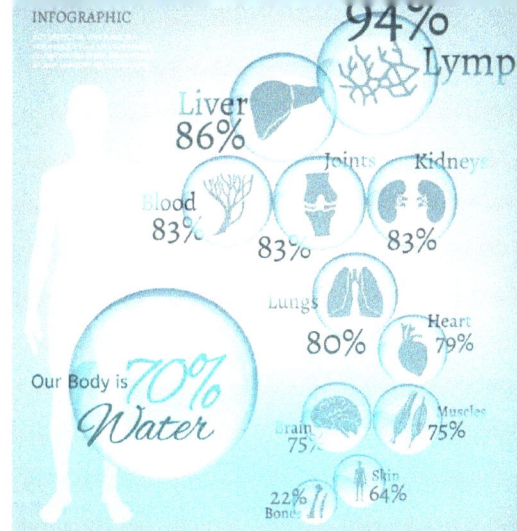

hormone additives can be helpful for some brains. I prefer buffalo because my system processes it very easily, but 3.5 oz. of raw, grass fed ground beef contains:

- 25% of RDA of B3
- 37% of RDA of B12 (which may not pass the blood-brain barrier in veggie sources)
- 18% of RDA for B6
- 32% of RDA for zinc
- 24% of RDA for selenium
- 12% of high quality, easier to absorb, heme iron

And 4 oz. of a grass fed raw bison patty contains:

- 34% of RDA of B12
- 26% of RDA of zinc
- 24% of RDA of selenium
- 22% of niacin
- 20% of B6
- 16% of iron
- 95mg of omega 3 fatty acids
- 653 mg of omega 6 fatty acids
- Numerous minerals including calcium, magnesium, phosphorus, & potassium
- And it has fewer calories, more protein and less fat than beef

Red meat is packed with nutrients that benefit the brain in many ways. It may not be right for everyone, but I've met several people who were previously vegetarians that began having health issues whose neurologist told them to begin eating red meat. Many of my earlier laxity and chronic spasm with inflammation issues resolved with the inclusion of red meat. Red meat was well received by my body right away in spite of not eating it for 20 years. Certain nutrients, particularly vitamins like K2 (MK4 in the brain), A, and B12 are more easily received from meat, as well as D3, iron, zinc, and iodine which are present in higher amounts in animal products. (Georgia Ede, MD; "*Your Brain on Plants: Micronutrients and Mental Health,* Diagnosis: Diet, December 2018)

Professional treatment options

There are many ways to recover from a head injury, and as mentioned earlier, a fall or accident can land differently in each person depending upon many factors. Taking it into consideration that each person might manifest a little differently with brain trauma, it could be helpful to be aware of the different types of rehabilitation approaches that are out there. Some treatment professionals include but are not limited to:

- Audiologists and Sound therapists (like Tomatis)
- Cognitive rehab therapists
- Chiropractors and Chiropractic neurologists
- Neuro-psychologists

- Occupational therapists
- Optometrists or Opthamologists (who practice color therapy)
- Physiatrists
- Physical Therapists and Manual therapists
- Nutritionists specializing in brain nutrition
- Speech therapists
- Exercise physiologists
- Functional medicine physicians
- Functional neurologists
- Osteopathic physicians
- Cranial Sacral Therapists
- Advanced Rolfers or Myofascial release practitioners
- Orientation and mobility therapists
- Lymphatic drainage
- Feldenkrais and Hanna Somatic Education
- NeuroMuscular Reeducation with Trigger Points and skin rolling
- Sensory integration specialist

There are a few scans available in some areas to get a better idea of which areas of the brain have been impacted, such as the PET scan, SPECT scan, and qSPECT (quantitative single photon emission computed tomography).New helmets have also been devised for football players that can provide information about the forces being applied in an impact to help determine whether or not the player should be taken out of the game. Although it's not the norm for someone to collapse and die from a single hit, it does happen and it's almost impossible to tell what happened inside someone's skull without a scan.

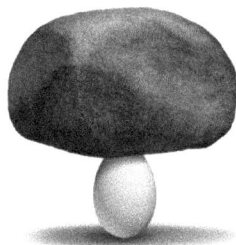

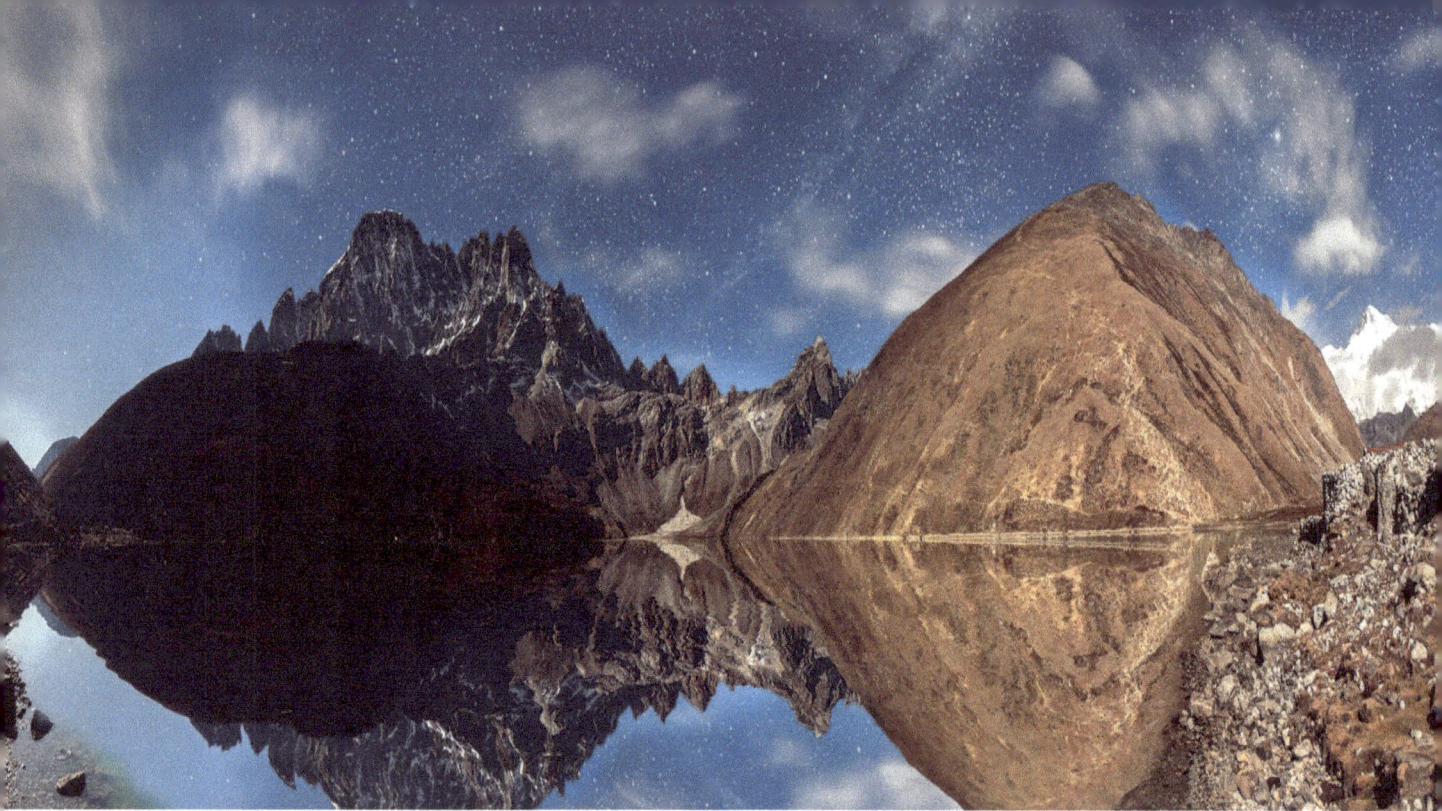

Chapter 5

The Awakening Body
and the Looking Glass

"Every human being is the author of his own health or disease.
To keep the body in good health is a duty… otherwise we shall not be able
to keep our mind strong and clear."
~ Buddha

This next chapter will be dedicated to a few safe exercises to do that can assist in reorganizing and retraining the brain. They'd be helpful whether there's been a head injury or not, since opening, awakening, and re-integrating the system feels amazing and useful for day-to-day aches and pains from stiffness, repetitive strain, sitting or standing for long periods, and injury recovery. It's also a plus for preventative maintenance to discourage the type of compressing, shearing, torqueing forces that can accumulate and create damage.

Identifying patterns

Deciding to take up bowling again late in life was one of the most significant and far-reaching choices I could have stumbled upon. It exposed some limitations that could easily be shifted, and the adventure of discovering how to remove them was life-altering. It not only served to wake up my body in that activity, but it extended to the other sports I was involved in as well. I was inspired to feel into what my pelvis was doing during the swing in racquetball, and how my foot was landing before the swing. Using my left hand suddenly became much easier and more forceful as something began to wake up in my right brain, and as my base and center of gravity became more stable.

In basketball I noticed that I turned towards the basket the same way every time I picked up the ball to shoot again, and remembered that the neurologist had asked me to turn a different way to go up the stairs or to head towards the kitchen so stimulate the side of the brain that had weakened. I began applying that to the game mainly to break up unconscious habits, but also to put my brain on alert while learning something new. The doctor had also suggested that I bounce the ball with the left hand, so I added that back in and continued to do it until I felt my brain respond.

Doing so actually brought my left brain on board instead of the right, perhaps because I was thinking about doing it differently? It was in the area of the motor cortex that I felt aliveness enter, so the goal of engaging more of my brain in order to awaken more of my body (and vice-versa) was being achieved. While swimming I noticed the residuals of the left-sided contraction all the way down through the torso from the injury where the pot fell on my head. That injury had created a frozen shoulder on that side, but most of the range of motion had already returned, so it was natural to suspect the latissimus dorsi as the culprit. I found the contraction was being generated by multiple structures including the kidneys and spleen, which were also affected during the injuries.

Releasing them with visceral manipulation opened the thorax on that side, supporting greater ease with the lats and quadratus lumborum. Working with several layers that includes several systems is usually the more thorough way to approach resolution. The Somatic exercises I'll be recommending will include modifications of yoga asanas, since they work so well together and are a familiar place to begin. They will influence the endoderm and ectoderm by adjusting the mesoderm – the layer that includes bony and soft tissue. By the way, the movements I described during the kingpin epiphany section getting to the bottom of the residuals corrected that lingering left side contraction.

The body is a tapestry

Before approaching these movements, it's important to view the system as an interwoven tapestry - a beautifully and intimately connected web of seamlessly streaming form and function. Then it's easier to grock the concept of moving something in your foot and being able to have an influence in your neck and on everything in between the two. There actually is an intimate proprioceptive connection between the feet and the neck. While moving through these somatic configurations, be sure to go slowly enough to be able to notice a little snag somewhere along the fabric that could cause it to bunch or pinch.

As soon as you notice that spot, rotate the limb nearest it internally, then externally, until you find the position that renders it the most neutral or smooth, then continue the motion. Come back to that area where you first felt the snag and see if it's still there; if it is even a little bit, then move the limb the other way and try the original movement again. For this set of movement explorations, we'll just use the directions of extension and flexion – or anterior and posterior, and side-bending. They're much less risky for discs, and will be more helpful in elongating the spine, the muscles, and the chains of fascia that may be pulling on the skull.

Remember that anything released on the lower body will serve the upper body and allow it to be more amenable to change. Addressing tensions around or inside the head while forces and contractions beneath it are still activated could make the pressures on the head and neck more uncomfortable. However, using movements that engage everything at the same time could be a safer way to explore initially. In any case, keep that in mind while doing stretches on your own at home. Always move slowly and gradually, to facilitate distinguishing as many sensations as you can. Eventually, if not right away you'll begin to feel relationships between areas in your body that need each other to be in sync for a full relaxation of the pattern to happen.

One pattern that's pretty reliable is the reciprocal one of the extensors and flexors. The flexors tend to be more engaged during daily life activities and will in time apply forces that strain structures on the back side. For example, the pectoralis muscles will be used quite a bit while working on the computer, doing dishes, cooking, etc. and will be straining the rhomboids in between the shoulder blades if not released. It's usually a good idea to open the areas that have been in the same position for long periods at the end of the day, so broadening the chest and extending the hip and knee flexors would follow a day of sitting all day. Hanging from a bar could oppose the force of gravity on the chest cavity and from the weight of the arms and shoulder girdle, but you'd need to ease into the hanging gradually with support. That being the case, we'll start opening the anterior first.

Opening the anterior of the body - standing

Comfy lunge A

- find a comfortable distance that doesn't strain your knees and raise your arms; the rear foot can be flat or on the balls of your foot
- take a deep breath, lift your ribs up then slowly drop them with the exhale
- with the breath, lift the rib cage and shoulder girdle gently, then lower them separately, first the ribs, then the shoulders
- repeat a few times, noticing where the snags or catches might be in the hips, belly, diaphragm, intercostal muscles, or abs
- When you find a snag, lean forward slightly into it, than side bend towards it and lift out again until you feel it lengthen with ease or releases without pulling on it

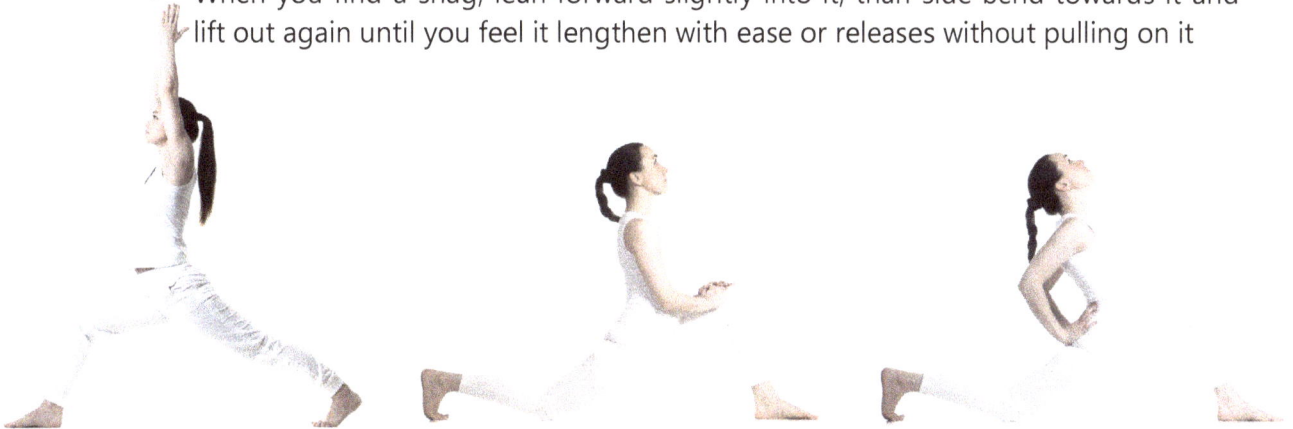

Comfy lunge B

- if your knees al ow, take a deeper stance and feel the line between the knee up through the thigh and into the abdomen; don't let knee go beyond foot
- pump the rear leg/foot up and down a bit and feel the influence on the
- change the angle of the rear leg in and out or lean forward slightly to see which one improves any tension along the chain
- lean back a little more only if it feels stable and sense the chain up through to the neck; make little adjustments to accommodate snags, if any

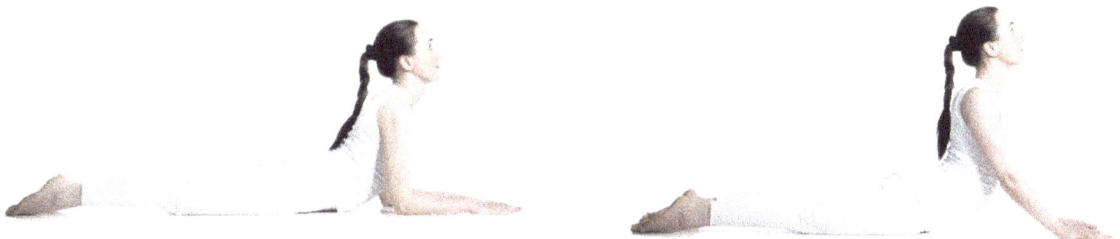

Opening the anterior of the body – lying down

Be sure that your neck tolerates extension before assuming this position. If you experience any difficulties, wait a couple of weeks and try it again. Whiplash injuries can create a tenderness in the neck that doesn't tolerate much extension or flexion, and whatever the case, please don't use analgesics to enable movements or positions that would otherwise not be workable. It's best to be able to feel where your body's at and respect its limitations while it's healing. There are modifications to be made so you can work up to varying degrees of extension.

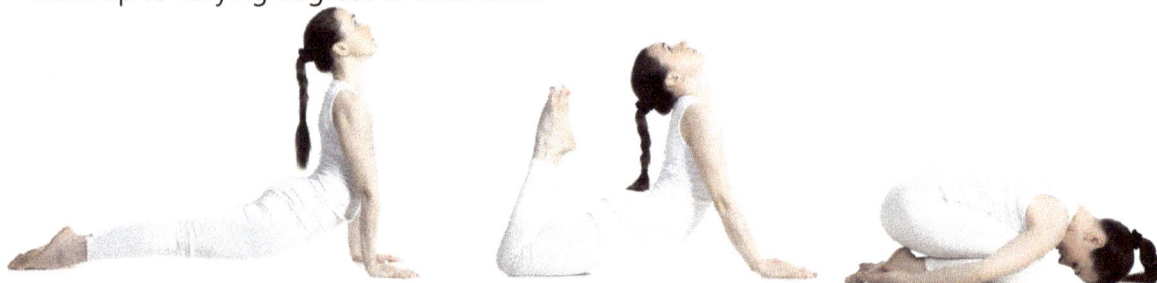

Pyramid and Cobra pose

- while lying face down, gently lift your head, neck, and chest until the arms are at a 45° angle and your nose is facing the floor
- slowly extend your head away from your neck and feel the soft traction down the spine to your sacrum
- come back to neutral with your head and gently extend one leg away from your waist, again feeling the pull reach up through the pelvis and spine
- then extend one leg and your head at the same time, feeling for any glitchy places along the path from your foot to your head
- slowly push up until your arms are at 90°, lift your head and neck until your eyes are facing forward and notice the line up through your sternum and neck, then feel if any snags appear in the throat area or ribs
- gradually lift and lower your head, raising and dropping your chin, feeling the traction up the anterior, then posterior sides of your body
- compare the right and left sides of your body with each position of the head, then make tiny adjustments in a side bend favoring the side with the snag, then come back to center and repeat the straight up and down move
- when the snags and glitches have been ironed out, straighten your arms if it feels comfortable to do so, lift your chest and extend the head again
- repeat the instructions above modifying for any snags in the chain from the feet to the head, such as slight side bend or flexion into the snag, hold, breathe, then lift and lengthen again
- look slightly left while sliding the right leg away from your pelvis as before,; look slightly right while sliding your left leg away, then come back down to the floor and rest in neutral position with your forehead on your hands
- if it feels comfortable, lift a little higher with your chest and head to increase the stretch through your torso and sense again where the pulls may be along the

frontal plane

- feel all the way down to the quads in your thighs, including where they attach at the upper parts of the femur
- flex down and back up slightly between the pelvis and diaphragm, allowing the abdominals to lengthen, sensing the effect on the thighs and chest
- bend your legs at the knee to increase the stretch even more if it feels easy, and extend your head to include the anterior cervical and throat area
- gently open and close your mouth, paying attention to the influence on your abdominal area, chest, and throat area
- make slight adjustments to your position to reduce any sense of a tightening along this length of fascial 'fabric', breathing into the area to supply a little more energy and awareness there
- slowly, gradually come out of the extension and work your way down to the floor, folding yourself over into a child's pose, if your joints allow
- if not, come back down to lie flat with your forehead on your hands and rest there in neutral position, taking stock of the sensations coursing through your system
- notice if there are areas that feel more vitalized than others and keep track as you repeat the movements to see if it equalizes, with the understanding that some areas may produce more sensation than others while healing

For any change in position after a head or brain injury you'll have to see what your system will tolerate. Using baby steps you can work your way back into just about any activity if you do so gradually and mindfully. Recovery takes quite a bit longer if you unwittingly re-injure yourself when you begin to feel better. It can require summoning more patience than you knew you had in some ways, along with compassion to quell the mounting frustrations you may feel as you hold off on some of your favorite activities. Modification is the best way to go so that you can find a way to participate with limitations.

For example, when my system was triggered into spasm by cold water, I'd go swimming in a half wet suit. When jumping jacks wouldn't work I'd use an elliptical machine instead to reduce the jarring impact. When I couldn't hear in busy restaurants I'd go during the slowest times, and shop when the least amount of people would be there to make it in and out as quickly as possible. Instead of playing racquetball for an hour or more, I'd play for fifteen minutes, and in dance class I'd restrict the planes of motion to the ones my spine could handle. If I was still getting dizzy in the sun I'd find a shady tennis court to play on, or wait until the temperatures were cooler. Phone conversations didn't go past 9:00 pm, and the television or radio went to half volume.

Practicing the modifications in these movements will help to dial in the sensitizing to what your body prefers, to which sensations are fine, and which need attention. There was period of time when I danced without rotating at all, and I stooped rather than bending over for quite a few months. I also changed how or whether I carried my purse or packages to alleviate pressures on the rib cage and thoracic outlet area, which also pulled on the neck. When a little more discernment is added to what the discomfort is, you don't feel overwhelmed or frustrated at how limiting an injury can be. Instead you feel liberated by the care, mindfulness, and learning it produces.

Now that all that's been covered, we can move into a more sensitive area that benefits greatly from being decompressed and opened out, but it also has to be done with much care and attentiveness. Once the anterior and posterior planes are freed up and desensitized, the other directions can be added much more smoothly. Try to notice whether you're feeling your skin, the muscles or other soft tissues, or the joints and bone. Practice first by stretching a finger using focusing on sensations in the skin, then move the finger with muscles and discern the difference. Last, sense what the bone feels like when you bend the finger as well as when you stretch it away from your hand. Making these distinctions will take you a long way with the other movements suggested here.

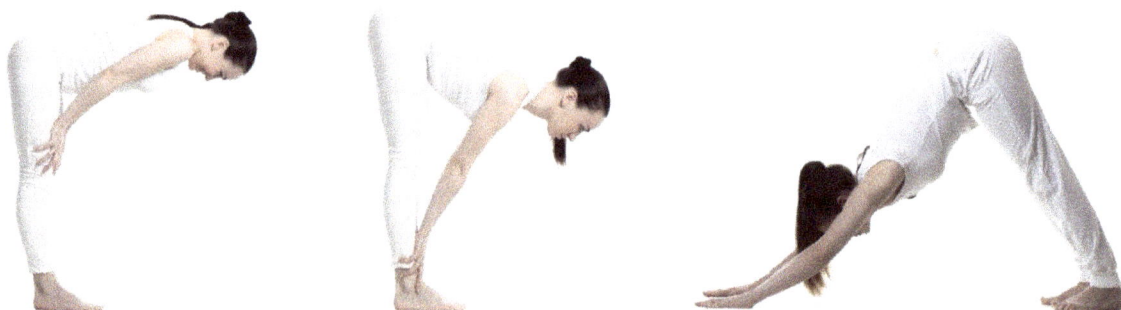

Opening the posterior of the body – standing
- as you begin to bend over, extend your torso away from your pelvis as though you're tractioning your spine, then extend your head away from your neck gently
- feel the rotation in your hip joints as you bend, because you're not bending at
- the waist, your rotating around the head of the femur – the thigh bone
- as you pull out and away from and through your spine, see if there are any sections or vertebrae that feel a little more stiff or sore than others
- if there are, make the smallest (about half an inch) side bend to the right at that segment, and the tiniest rotation, then come straight again then side bend to the left and return to center
- if it still feels a little stiff, you can do a tiny flexion and extension just at that segment if you can isolate to that degree, inhaling with the arch or extension, and exhaling with the curl, or flexion

- usually that will produce a release, but if it doesn't, it may well be a vertebrae above or below it, so repeat for the adjacent vertebrae
- come up if it begins to get uncomfortable; relax and shake it out, then start again later in the day
- work your way down gradually, checking for comfort at each vertebrae, and if you can, sense more deeply into and beneath the vertebrae into the canal where the spinal cord and dura are; or you can picture them
- there are also anterior and posterior longitudinal ligaments alongside the vertebral column that respond by softening if you put your attention there

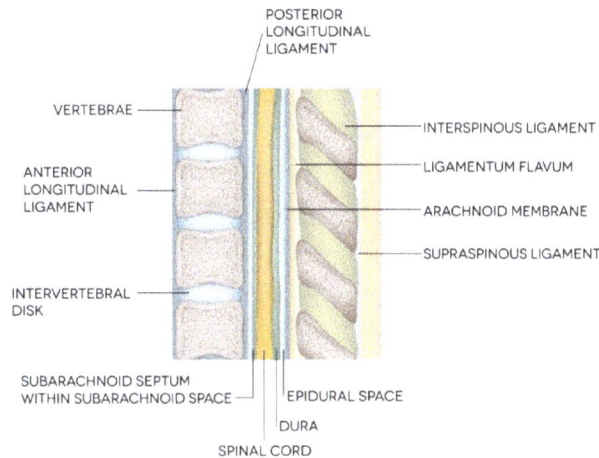

POSTERIOR LONGITUDINAL LIGAMENT

VERTEBRAE

ANTERIOR LONGITUDINAL LIGAMENT

INTERVERTEBRAL DISK

INTERSPINOUS LIGAMENT

LIGAMENTUM FLAVUM

ARACHNOID MEMBRANE

SUPRASPINOUS LIGAMENT

SUBARACHNOID SEPTUM WITHIN SUBARACHNOID SPACE

EPIDURAL SPACE

DURA

SPINAL CORD

Using the continuum to rebalance the body

Bones can easily be displaced or compressed by the connective tissue all around them, and the soft tissue surrounding the skeleton can easily contract and become irritated by displaced or compressed bones. Muscles, ligaments, and tendons morph into bone by way of the periosteum so there's a continuum between the softer and denser structures in our bodies. Fascia not only envelopes muscles, but it also permeates them and provides a network of support. Not only is there continuity between muscles, connective tissue, and bones, but there is also continuity between blood vessels, lymphatic vessels, and nerve fibers, all of which interface with bones and soft tissue.

In this gestalt you can imagine how a pinched vessel or nerve fiber can irritate and contract soft tissue and how adhesions in soft tissue can entrap nerves, restrict blood flow, and stagnate the lymph flow. The posterior ipsilateral fascia and ligament streams from the inferior end of the body attach and/or intersect at the pelvis, then run up across the sacrum and up the spine to the skull where forces can be applied to the brain or into the face. In the same way happenstance forces in the face, as with braces, can cause pressure throughout the head and neck, which can generate superior to inferior tension in other areas of the body.

There are several layers of muscles on the back, many of them overlapping with a broad influence from the thighs, hips and shoulders. Some of the deeper layers that are adjacent to the spine, like the multifidus and longissimus travel all the way up to the head. A few of the more surface muscles in regular use by the shoulders, like the levator scapulae and trapezius, reach the upper region of the neck. I can safely say that practically all of the muscles in the back and shoulders that have a connection to the neck or head are intimately involved in a concussion or brain injury due to a fall, often neatly squared off in a quadrant as per the neurology.

In these cases, much more ease can come into the neck and shoulders by balancing the brain in its membranes, releasing dural tension, and settling excessive charge in brain nuclei. I've seen it help a great deal on tension from daily life stress as well. During a whiplash or a when an object falls on the top of the head, the force travels down the length of the back, usually capturing the posterior line nearest the core, down to or through the tailbone, crossing the lateral ligaments in the pelvic floor, and following nerve or meridian pathways all the way to the feet. Due to the overlapping tapestry of tissues, an irritation can easily spread to an adjacent area.

Head injuries will almost always insult cranial and cervical nerves, which will install pain and contractions in the face, chest, shoulder joint and girdle. Between the vagus, phrenic, greater occipital, subclavian nerves and brachial plexus, practitioners and patients alike can wind up boggled as to how to resolve the injury completely. Using movements that employ many of the major muscle groups while also using mini-movements that target sensory cells in and around the face and throat, the joints, vertebrae, and extremities can greatly contribute. Ample networks of connective tissue can also help settle and reorganize injured areas using self-applied myofascial methods. If you're not sure if a nerve is irritating a muscle or a muscle is impinging a nerve, go indirect rather than working directly on the sensitive area. Selecting global, gentle movements along with myofascial, neurovascular, cranial sacral, and lymphatic approaches that can reach through the tapestry and take advantage of its cross-talk.

A brain injury incorporates the endoderm (brain and nervous system) as well as the ectoderm (skin) layers predominantly, which could be why the skin rolling and trigger point work was so beneficial. Muscle tension in the mesoderm in my case happened as a by-product of nerve irritation and compression, rather than being a primary factor. In certain areas the subcutaneous nerves were connected to other nerve groups just like the superficial fascia led naturally into the mesoderm layers so that the impacts were widespread and the symptoms can be difficult to track. I was inspired to track them though, and spoke of what I found in more detail in the kingpin section a little later on.

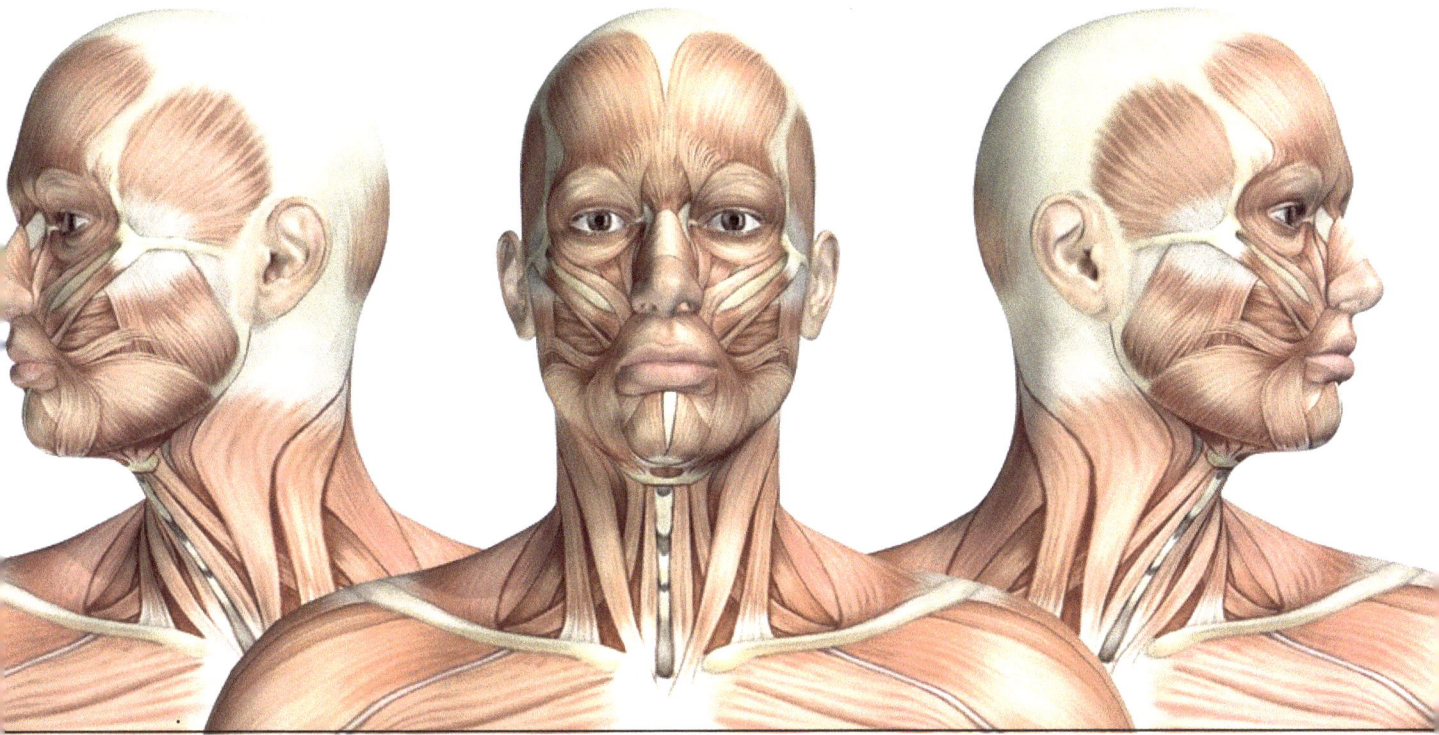

In summary, global affects local

For brain injuries to fully resolve, therefore, it seems using methods that message all three layers and also address the key nerve, visceral, and fluid systems within them would be the most useful in the long run. Depending upon the extent of the injury, a multi-discipline approach may be needed that includes life skills (occupational therapy) retraining and psychological support, along with cognitive rehabilitation or sensory integration methods. That said, some cognitive deficits, spatial, or balance issues as well as personality changes can and do reset when the brain heals. Only a small percentage of very severe brain injuries or the repeated, mild and moderate head traumas that aren't treated have symptoms that persist or get worse over time.

In most cases, brain nutrition, brain exercises, and aerobic exercise account for a huge percentage of that healing process, particularly in the endoderm. Some aspects of the dysregulation that follows head injuries correct with time, rest, and proper facilitation (brain stimulation), but others in the mesoderm layer respond well to manual therapy and neuromuscular reeducation. Dr. Hanna stated that, "A muscle can't respond to a conscious and unconscious message at the same time." So using mindful movements to bring those layers of contracted soft tissue back into coherence through cortical control can greatly reduce pain and spasm that might otherwise takes years to sort out. Particularly in the instances where brain dysregulation is the source of the issue, neuromuscular approaches can often be the most helpful. Although a hands-on session will attend to and reliably release local contractions, when released in context with the whole the results will be more lasting since it avoids the marginalized tail pulling the whole elephant back into the room.

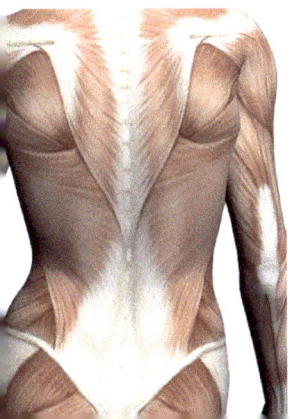

A significant amount of the information exchange that happens in conscious, whole body movements will also open energetic channels, stimulate fluid systems, and help bony displacements. Yet it's probably a good idea to visit a manual therapist fairly early on to have an assessment and manipulation of specific fluid and internal organ, nerve, and blood vessel lesions or cranial/brain deformations. If in doubt, there are several scan and assessment methods out there that can better pinpoint specific deficits and needs. After that, the exercises you do at home can account for the largest percentage of your recovery. You can feel empowered not only to share with your therapist what you've discovered in self-sensing, but also in taking care of much of the rehabilitation on your own. Not only will it then be assured to be tailored to your needs, but you'll also learn so much in the process.

Avoiding setbacks

What you do as well as what you modify or leave out of your day will all play an important role in the recovery being swift and complete. There will be times when stress is a little high or sleep is in short supply that some of the symptoms return briefly, but those times can also be an indicator of how far along you are in the healing process. As your system gets stronger, you can do more and more with less and less triggering of symptoms. Remember that doing too much just when you begin to feel better, particularly if you're still taking supplements or meds to reduce pain signals, could be giving your system the wrong message and provoke a setback the next day. **Tip #13**: Consider having an evening ritual that facilitates settling your system so that sleep comes more easily. Stretching and taking a bath before bed can often help a great deal.

How the injury sets up in your system will be unique in many ways, so it's always helpful to pay attention to which activities preceded a setback and take note on which symptoms turned up as a result. There may be adhesions from old injuries, surgeries, or genetic predispositions that play a part in how forces from impacts land in or shape your system. Remember that dropping into a still, quiet place in meditation can boost cognitive functioning, clarity, and focus, and provides the type of rest you'd receive during sleep. Meditation settles the nervous system and cultivates laughter and compassion, which includes compassion towards yourself. Being light-hearted about life events is in itself supportive of healing.

Take care in your movement sequences initially to work on one plane at a time, going inch by inch, testing how your body tolerates it. Make modifications along the way to capture and release the snags. Start slowly with the anterior and posterior planes, then include side bending or rotation movements. You can add them in combination when each plane is well tolerated. Consider modifying types and timing of activities for female athletes along with appropriate joint support. Consider researching the many professionals

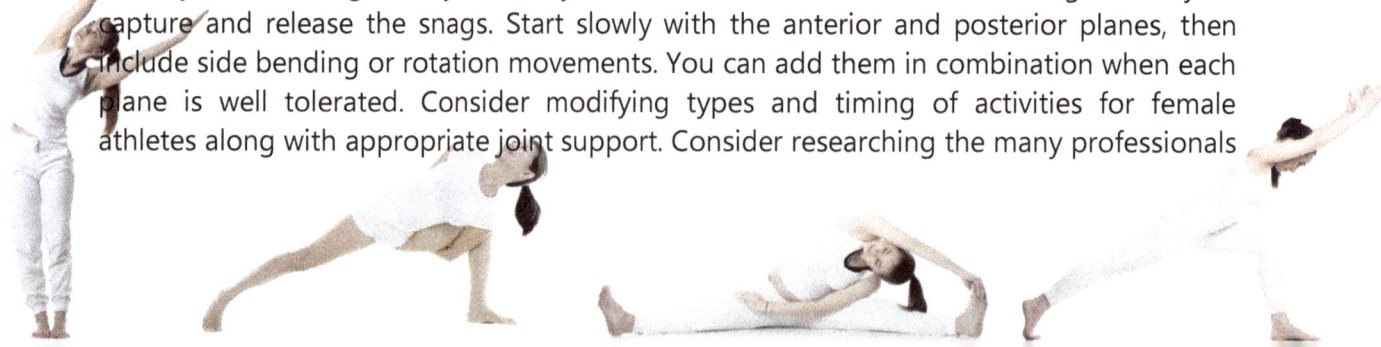

in your area who would be able to assist and help restore proper brain function, as well as advise you on how to maintain brain health on your own. These days you can check online to see who's in your area. There are many great practitioners who specialize in head and brain injury who can make a huge difference for you.

If a hot, clumsy mess like me can overcome 30 plus brain injury symptoms after repeated head trauma, I hope you feel encouraged and inspired that there's always potential to improve. Conscious awareness of your body facilitates a synchronous integration that feels like it counters the effect of gravity. When the system is opened, balanced, and integrated in a whole body way, the energies that flow through it are freed to do the work of carrying you around instead of muscular effort. A sign that integration is needed is often a sense of heaviness in the limbs or head, or a fatigue that sets in just holding yourself upright.

Include activities in your day that don't reproduce the pain signal, which is almost always a setback in itself. TENS units are used by physical therapists to reroute pain signals or help block them, and they can also be useful for some people. Versions of those units are available for home use. Get to know what your body doesn't handle well while it's in recovery and adhere to those boundaries. Plan for a little boost moment each day that you know is something you'll look forward to that makes you smile and lifts your spirits. Engage your mind in something all-consuming that you enjoy like a hobby or a fun project. It helps to bring in something to switch the tracks when your brain starts to slip. It changes how you relate to those symptoms so you don't become overwhelmed, helps you make better decisions within uncertainty, and also helps to remodel the brain.

The role of consciousness
There were awakenings in consciousness for me that did remain as access to some other layers of the intelligent, vast, field of possibilities that served my rehabilitation process. The layers include a space underneath the mind that prevents negative chatter in the brain from taking hold, and a place to be without thinking at all. Turning towards those other layers or dimensions of consciousness can settle you into a place that is subtler and therefore relieving to any structure, function, pattern, predisposition, pain distribution, thought process, background, or history. In fact, many times pain would disappear so fast that it made me wonder what was really creating it. Stress is a significant contributor to all types of inflammatory processes, imbalances and tension in your system, which can be undone in large part by meditative, mindful, or contemplative practices.

Leaning into other layers of consciousness opens a field of altruism, love, and joy or bliss that makes whatever pains or challenges life may present much less traumatic. There's immense value in not having the manifestations of a traumatic injury destroy the quality of your daily life interactions, even in the midst of the most off-balance times. That type of awareness can cut through a field of fog and allow a ray of clarity that helps you continue to discern, unpack, and design a treatment protocol for yourself. The brain does a much better job for you if things are resolved so that energy and attention are freed up to be directed towards maintaining or reestablishing balance. Settling into a different layer in consciousness with meditation frees that energy up. Having a resolution ritual at the end of the day whereby outstanding odds and ends of plans or thought processes are finalized. Thinking it through in the shower or in a journal gives the body and mind rest and supports having a better night's sleep, and so does discharging the senses by staring into a night sky.

Like anything, meditation gets easier with practice. Setting aside fifteen or twenty minutes here and there each day or each week to tune into a silent place inside, to look at the space in between thoughts, or to just sit under a redwood tree in the forest, prepares you for easy access to the space in more difficult times. Consciousness, in other words, can be a valuable ally in life in general, but also in recovery from traumatic injury. Contemplation alone can achieve a level of integration that facilitates opposing gravity, but so does being as consciously present in as aware as possible of the sensations in your body. You'll feel so different when you stand up or move it'll be like having a brand new body all over again each time you maintain that presence in the tissue fields.

When the principles behind what makes Biodynamic Cranial work or Feldenkrais movements effective are employed, there exists a form of contemplation as one turns his or her awareness to the movement of life and the forces that enable that movement to occur. That contemplation will include the awareness of the palpable presence that flows from a Higher intelligence into and through form, ever creating and recreating itself in endless expressions that can be as precise and intricate as also chaotic and mysterious. What founder A. T. Still's prodigy, W. Sutherland described as the system's Primary Respiration mechanism sums it up neatly: *"It is a functional mechanism that manifests from the implicate order to the explicate order in the tissues, bring nutrition to the cell and carrying metabolic wastes away. It comes from that which precedes everything, that which is primary, that is, the Love of God, which exists in the implicate order, manifesting the breath of air in the explicate order."* (R. Paul Lee, DO; Interface, 2005)

The importance of movement, particularly the movement of fluids is where the Breath of Life enters and is expressed is through all systems. Without fluids no other structure could function. *"The potency of the fluids is mandatory for life according to Sutherland. "CSF (cerebrospinal fluid), blood, lymph, extracellular and intracellular fluids carry this divine nourishment, information, and knowledge from the Mind of God." (Lee, 2005)*

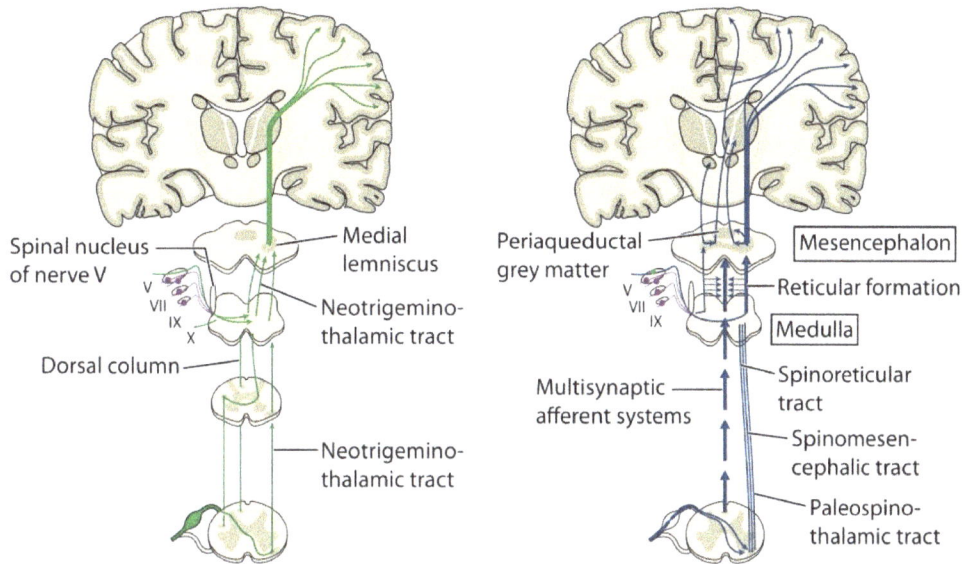

Spinal nucleus of nerve V — Medial lemniscus — Neotrigemino-thalamic tract — Dorsal column — Neotrigemino-thalamic tract

Periaqueductal grey matter — Mesencephalon — Reticular formation — Medulla — Multisynaptic afferent systems — Spinoreticular tract — Spinomesen-cephalic tract — Paleospino-thalamic tract

For the sensitive and savvy

During one of my osteopathic sessions I could feel that something the doctor was doing on my head sent a sensation down my spine to the tailbone. I felt the release through the entire length of the dural tube. One other time she was working on top of the cranium on a sore spot, I felt the release into the legs, giving me the impression she had influenced the descending pathways, perhaps using the corticospinal tract since it's so large and long. You can use the image above as a reference, but it doesn't include the many areas of the midbrain or brainstem that the pathways cross and pass through, nor are all of the pathways included. It just gives you a visual to help imagine where it's happening.

I decided to try contacting these structures on my own one day, and low and behold, the involuntary postural muscles released as did the erector spinae. Each time I used it on my clients the same thing happened so I felt I was really influencing those descending pathways also, but by contacting the midbrain just above the inion, which is probably how the involuntary set was influenced. In my own body I listened for sensations from the brain nuclei as buzz, charge, agitation, the sound of wind, or running water, or a high pitched sound, and began to make associations. There are also many tender areas on my skull. Making light contact with the tender or buzzy area would always relax the paraspinals.

Possibly the ascending pathways were also being affected, settling down the feedback which altered the excitation of the feedforward part of the loop. This made me curious about the somatosensory cortex, which must have been the area where the doctor was working, although she may have had a different intent. I checked the body map on the homunculus and worked near the central sulcus (midline) area where the hips and legs can be influenced. The size of the body part gives you an idea of how much of the brain is dedicated to its function.

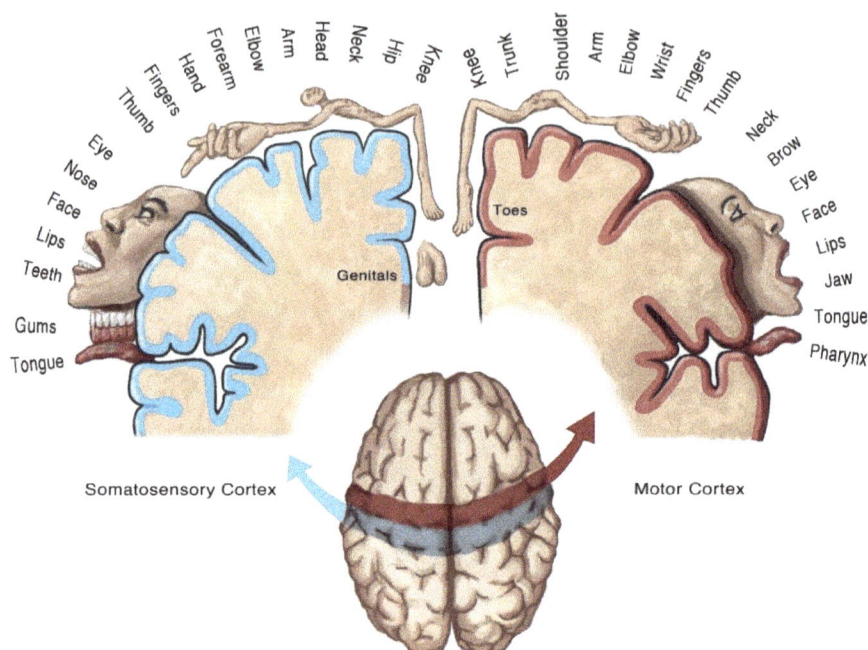

Somatosensory Cortex   Motor Cortex

As a test, while I was on a walk the other day I noticed my left hip felt higher than the right and also had some sensation of tension and soreness around the greater trochanter. While continuing to walk I made gentle contact with the middle of the top of my head where nerve signals for the hips are located, slightly anterior for motor pathways, and the hip corrected itself; it balanced. In other instances I found that the contractions were settled more by working with the posterior thalamus through which sensory information is relayed. The next experiment was to hold the thalamus (through intention) area and sensory-motor cortex on the central sulcus at the same time while walking. Not only did the sensations in the hip diminish, but the soreness in my right ankle did as well. In the case of the ankle, the sore spot on the cranium corresponded to that of the ankle.

It's impossible to tell exactly what's going on as you offer input into the system, but one thing is for sure: it's responding. If you're game to combine movement while contacting the sensory motor cortex, find a comfortable place to lie down and begin searching for spots of tension that feel co-created by paired joints. Work up from your foot, ankle, knee, hip, pelvis, thorax, shoulder and neck, like in the exercises described earlier, combining two or three areas. Put them in a position of ease with rotation, side-bending, flexion, or extension. Go further into that ease as the areas soften while placed in slack. Place your hand (s) on the sides of your head, or between the vertex and the inion and discover which area enhances the release.

Then gently come out and rediscover which combined position places them in maximum tension, and wait for the softening. In my system, while the ankle is dorsi-flexed and the hip is in external rotation for ease, holding the thalamus or claustrum area, they both soften even more. In the tension direction of plantar flexion and internal rotation of the hip, they also soften, while holding at the cortex was neutral.

Using the throat and mouth to release the brain

Several structures inside the mouth, above the nose, under the tongue, under the chin, in the throat and behind the jaw connect to membranes or bones that impact the brain. For that reason, using gentle stretches that involve the jaw, the tongue, face, and ears can relieve pressures from the brain and even release pain. They can be one of the most affected areas that take longest to resolve due to how deep they are, so direct access will be limited. Falls or blunt forces to the back or front of the head will inevitably land in the throat. The soft tissue connections transmit these forces in every direction to the eyes, ears, skull, esophagus, heart, ears, neck, and brain.

The other potential injury which is very common in head injuries, including whiplash, is the loss of the cervical curve. The curves in the spine are excellent shock absorbers that protect the spine as well as the brain from the impacts that travel up the skeleton just from walking, jumping, running, or climbing – most any weight-bearing activity. So whenever that curve is compromised or lost, it propels additional forces into areas that are already vulnerable to damage from wear and tear. It is something that can be fixed, but valuable to know about and watch out for. Even lying on a rolled up towel for twenty minutes a day can help substantially.

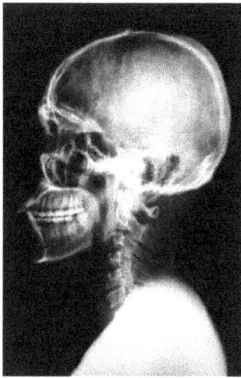

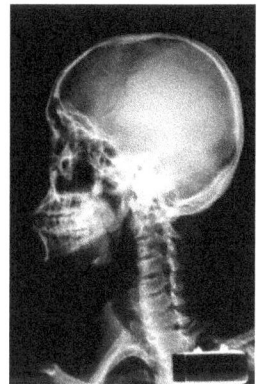

Fascial connections will often play a huge role in how and where to treat lingering issues from head injuries, including those in the throat. The lack of glide will make those restrictions easy to spot. Sometimes the treatment will need to be fairly specific when it's a key area of strain or damage, and if you know which areas are most likely to hold the impact, it'll save you a lot of time and discomfort. Chiropractic or basic massage will not automatically release this web of influences. Injury is one area where specificity goes a long way. When an accident happens, your whole body hits the ground, and with a whiplash your entire spine gets flailed around. So treating the entire spine initially in a more general way, and addressing all the fluid fields will be a tremendous help. The next steps then would lie in locating the particular spinal segment, or the adjacent ligament, the torsion in the meninges, the organ firing back into a nerve, the restricted vessel adjacent to the nerve, and so on, for the web of complexity to resolve.

The most superficial layer of fascia that connects the thorax, neck and head is the platysma. It is a wide band of fascia originating from the entire span across the pectoralis in the chest, the deltoids in the shoulder, crossing the clavicle, then runs up the neck to insert along the jaw line and muscles of the face. It is bound to receive and transmit the shock of collision forces into the face and skull as well as throughout the delicate thoracic outlet area where several nerves and blood vessels must pass. Although underneath the platysma, the most superficial layer of the deep cervical fascia is called the investing layer. It wraps around the neck like a collar, attaching to the hyoid bone in the throat, the scapula, clavicle, and manubrium, as well as across the superior nuchal line like the upper trapezius, down to the nuchal ligament of the spine. There is a deeper anterior layer of fascia that surrounds the esophagus, thyroid gland, trachea, and infrahyoid muscles.

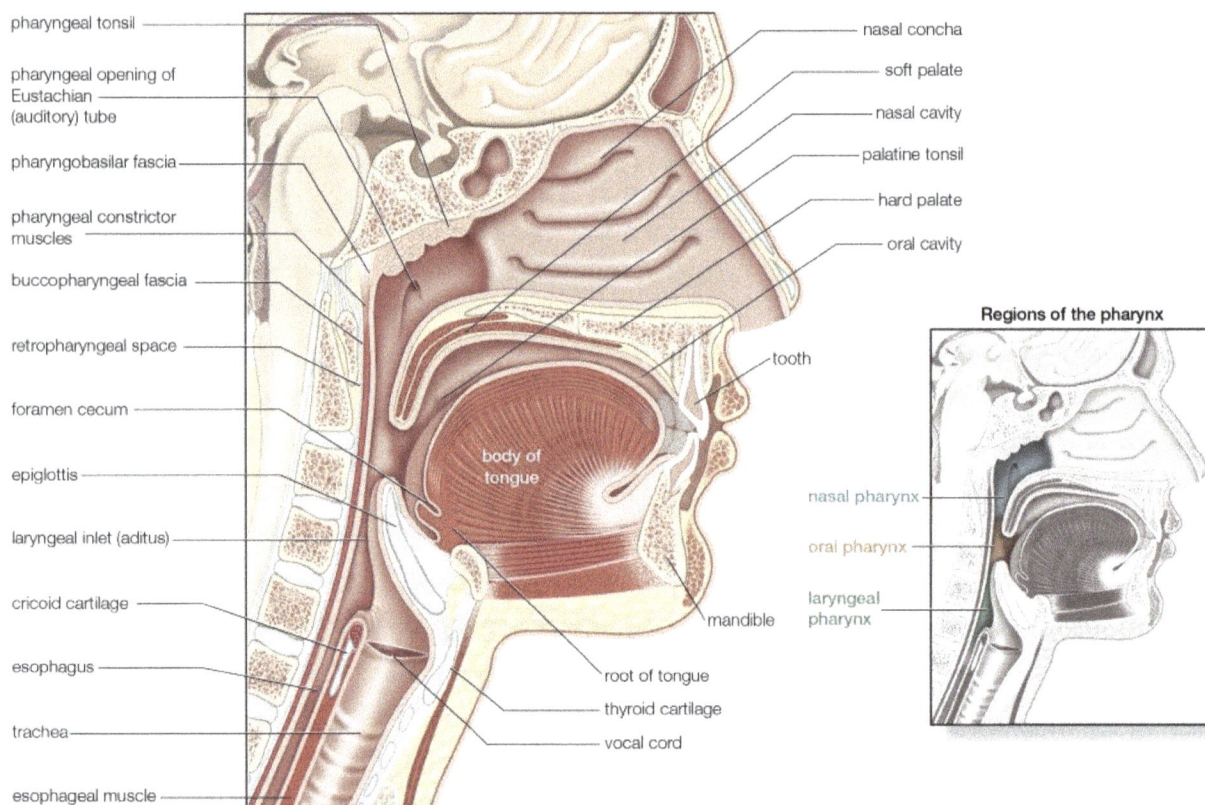

Regions of the pharynx

This layer connects with the buccopharyngeal fascia behind the tongue and so can be indirectly accessed by contacting its most inferior attachments while moving the tongue and mandible. The deepest fascia layer is the prevertebral fascia that is surrounding your vertebral column and its musculature, prevertebral muscles, deep back muscles, and scalenes. It runs from the base of the skull down through the spine attaching to the spinous, nuchal ligament and transverse processes as well as the fascia of the rib cage. The carotid sheath, which surrounds the carotid artery, jugular vein, vagus nerve, and cervical lymph nodes, are also connected to all the other deeper fascia layers. Needless to say, this is a key layer of tissue that can have a tremendous impact throughout the head, neck, shoulder, and thoracic areas, which is not separate from fascial chains down through the hips and legs. We'll approach it through adjacent structures using movement.

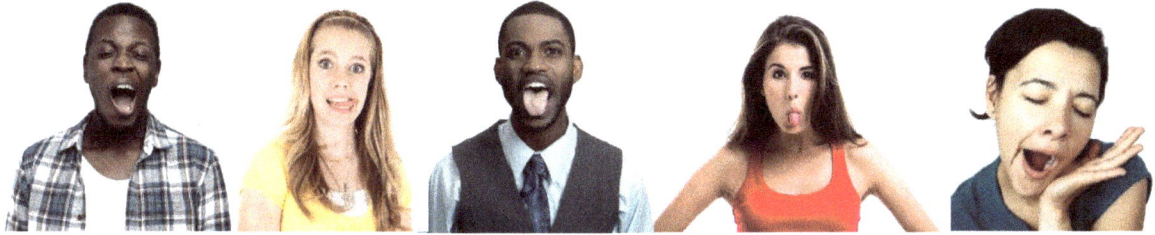

Exercises using the jaw and tongue

Many of the most tender areas after head trauma lie in these deeper layers of fascia, which also generate several trigger points. A way to reach them can be through the soft tissue relationships at the back of the mouth that are replete with sensory organs that will clarify which layer, or which side of the structure feels the most tense or irritated. Now that you have a better idea of what and where these structures in the mouth, throat, and neck are, you can get a better picture of what is being contacted when you use these movements. The brain is very visual and will be responsive to you visualizing the area if not the exact structures you would like to influence or release. Just know that as you move your jaw and tongue you will be accessing the back of your throat and those connections around the back of your head. You'll also touch into areas around your spine, blood vessels, lymph, nerves, glands, and relevant muscles, cranial bones and membranes to release pressures on the brain.

The sphenoid bone, which attaches to every other bone inside your skull, also connects to a membrane that runs through the center of your brain. Your lower jaw, or mandible, will be moving structures inside your mouth that can access that inner layer of fascia behind the tongue, but will

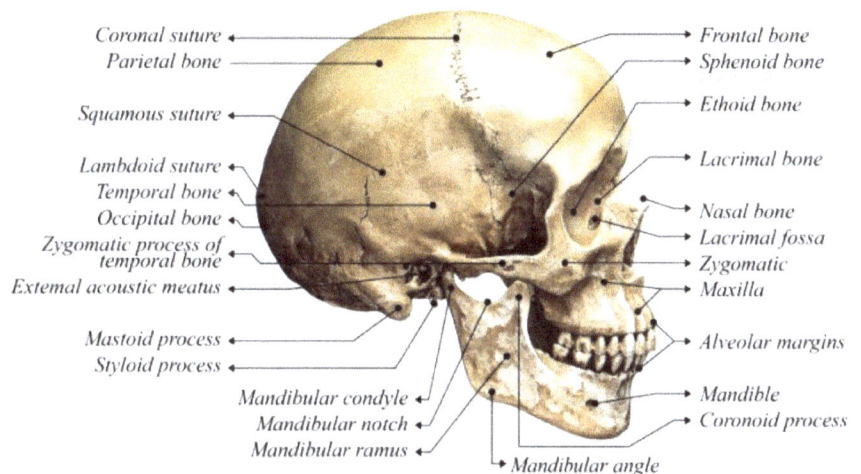

Coronal suture
Parietal bone
Squamous suture
Lambdoid suture
Temporal bone
Occipital bone
Zygomatic process of temporal bone
External acoustic meatus
Mastoid process
Styloid process
Mandibular condyle
Mandibular notch
Mandibular ramus
Frontal bone
Sphenoid bone
Ethoid bone
Lacrimal bone
Nasal bone
Lacrimal fossa
Zygomatic
Maxilla
Alveolar margins
Mandible
Coronoid process
Mandibular angle

also reach the maxilla, zygomatic arch, and vomer which all reach into the interior fascial layers. Initially, just move your jaw around from side to side, up and down to see how free it feels. Don't do this if you know you have TMJ whereby you hear or feel your jaw joint popping when you open your mouth. Notice if the jaw wants to drift to one side. Turn your attention to the base of your skull and feel the connection as you open and close your mouth. Then flex and extend your neck, lifting your chin up, then down towards your chest. In each direction extend your lower jaw away from your neck as if there was an overbite with the bottom teeth. Then swivel your mandible (lower jaw) to the left, feeling the subtle stretch for the masseter and behind your ears near the mastoid bone.

Next, tilt your head at an angle while moving and jutting out your jaw and locate the areas and positions that reveal the restrictions. Breathe into them while moving back and forth in the opposite direction, then back to the tight area a few times to let it reorganize. Come back to center and this time use your tongue instead of your mandible. Stick it out in different directions while sensing the influence at the sub-occipital area. Flex, extend, tilt, and side-bend your head while exploring different positions with your tongue, sensing and releasing tensions inside your mouth and at the base of your skull if not inside around the brain stem and cerebellum. Consider using mini-movements so you can discern the point at which a change in sensation happens. Reverse directions if you hit a tender zone, then come back to it after moving freely for as long as you can in the opposite direction.

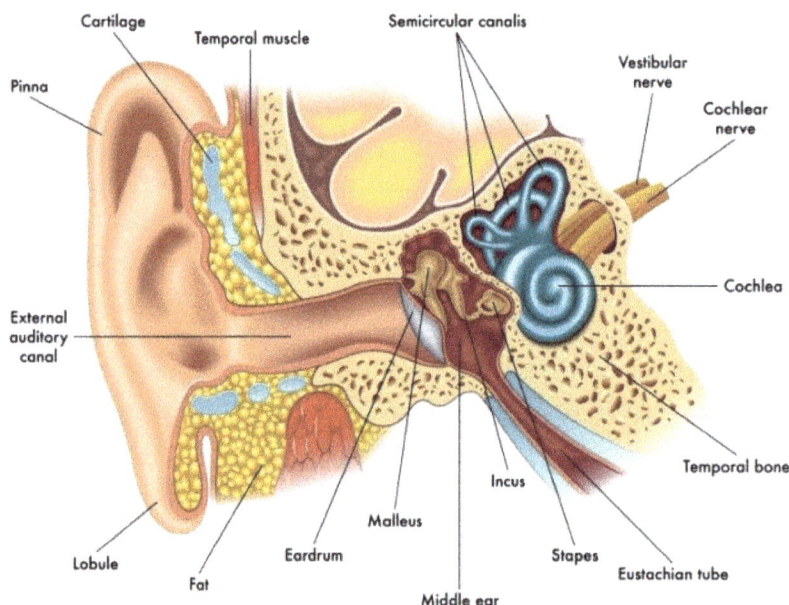

Releasing pressures using the ears

The physical ears can have an effect on the temporal bone that is adjacent to the pinna, or outer ear. The Eustachian tube in the middle ear connects with the throat, and Dr. Michael Burcon reported in 2006 that there is also an intimate connection with the upper cervical area and the ears. Vertigo and tinnitus, often experienced in brain injury, along with Meniere's disease have all been able to resolve by treating the upper cervical and sub-occipital areas, as have migraines and ear infections.

Whenever approaching an area of your body recently affected by an injury, it's best to go slowly and very gently. For this exercise it's best to wait until the pain has subsided before trying it, as it touches into areas that are intimately involved in head trauma. After the acute phase, it can be very helpful in removing residual strain and tension patterns that could become ongoing triggers. It can also be used as a type of preventive maintenance as the tendency may remain for these areas to tighten up when over-stimulated, even by sound. It's just as easy to become sensitized to sound as it is to visual stimuli. Over-stimulation has a tendency to generate tinnitus – ringing in the ears – headaches or neuralgia, and fatigue.

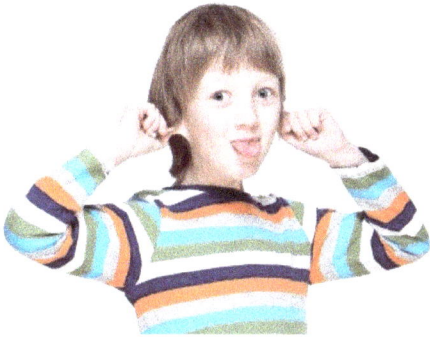

Start by holding the helix of the outer ear, a little higher up than the lobes. Extend out and down gently, noticing which side seems tighter as you visualize the temporal bone on the other side of the skin. Hold lightly until you feel the tighter side let go, then stick out your tongue and tilt your head if needed to support the release of the throat tensions that can be accessed with the ears. Touch one finger with another, just barely touching the skin on each finger. That's the lightness of pressure and gentleness needed to move these delicate structures and sense their responses. Try fluttering your lips using the 'horse lips' at the same time and feel the opening near the brain stem.

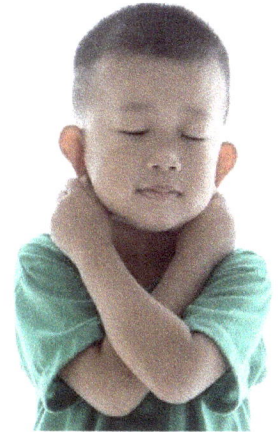

Working directly with the cranium

Another key area that has a great affect is the bridge of the nose that connects to the ethmoid bone which, through the glabella and smaller crista galli bone, connects to the falx and sphenoid mentioned earlier that is attached to every bone in your skull. The weight of reading or sunglasses can apply pressures to these tender areas while they're healing, so using the lightest possible pair helps. This significant crossroads also affects the falx cerebri which intersects the brain as well as the tentorium, in addition to being almost exactly where the entry point to the bladder meridian sits.

Blood vessels that branch off from the external carotid artery rest there, along with the junction of the frontal bone with the upper aspect of the eye socket. Gentle pressure here can be immensely relieving, and you might the upper corners a little tender or sensitive. If so, move your fingers up into the little divot just beneath the inner curve of the eyebrows, which will be bladder 2. Press and release here a few times before returning to the point adjacent to the tear ducts. You may feel a release that extends all the way down your back following the length of the meridian to your feet.

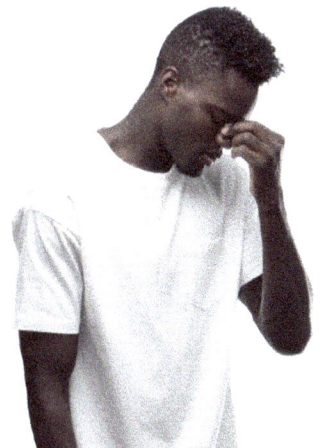

Frontal bone — Coronal suture
Parietal bone — Forehead boss
Supraorbital process — Glabella
Temporal bone — Supraorbital foramen
Nasal bone — Sphenoid bone
Lacrimal bone
Zygomatic bone — Ethmoid bone
— Maxilla
— Volmer
Nasal concha — Nasal spine
Aveolar process — Ramus
— Angle of jaw
Mandible — Mental protruberance
Mental tuberosity — Mental protruberance

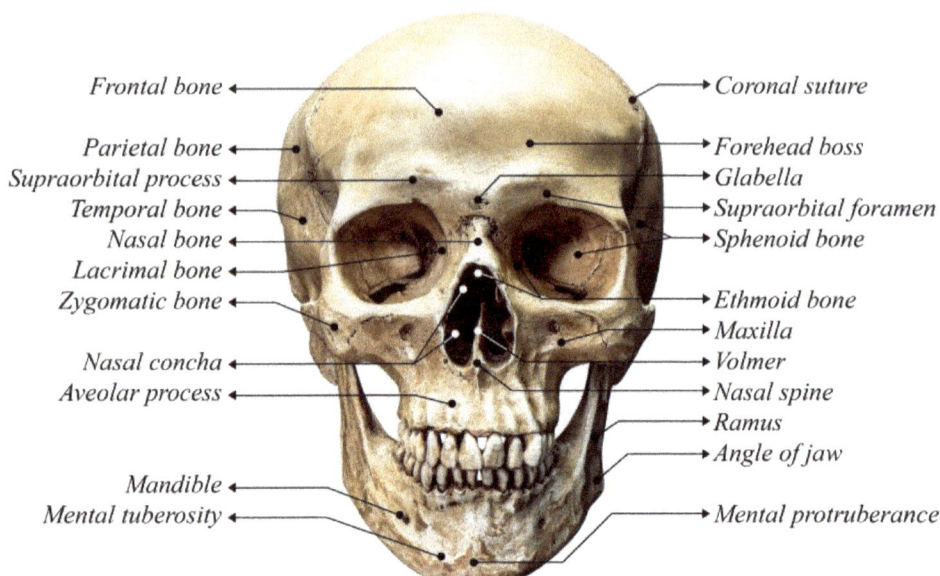

Because the sphenoid also has dural connections that attach to the meninges that surrounds the spinal cord, it has potential to relax the entire spine. The eyes share some neural connections with the tentorium cerebelli by way of the greater occipital nerve right at C2. The falx intersects the tentorium cerebelli at the cranial base, so whatever may influence the balance of one of these membranes can also shift tensions in the other, which will affect both the neck and the eyes. It's not uncommon for neck tension to release by balancing these inter-cranial membranes.

Once you get the feel for it, you can begin to tell which side of the falx feels tighter or more tender, then stick out your tongue and check to see if it corresponds to the side of mouth that also holds more tension. Move your tongue over in the opposite direction of the tighter side while holding the bridge of your nose and you should feel a release in the mouth, jaw, neck, and eyes. There are several rectus capitus muscles just underneath the skull in the front and back of the head that attach it to the neck. The posterior rectus capitus are reflexive with the eyes. These ten little muscles will surely be tightened with impacts to the head. They are deeply seated right next to the bone, so in order to access them with movement, you'll want to make very small articulations with your head. Your head is pressing into your hand, not the other way around.

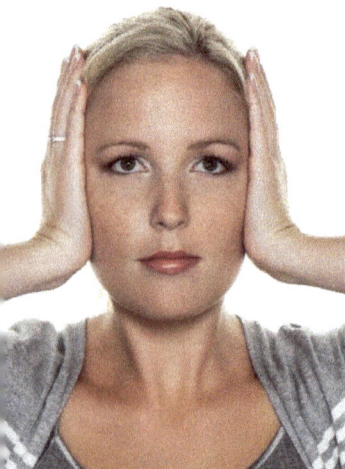

It's a tiny, muscle energy micro movement that will engage these muscles slightly, then release them in the opposite direction just a bit. Less is more. You can start in the flexion/extension direction, pressing gently forward about an inch into your hand that's resting on your forehead, then release backwards an inch and a half. Switch your receiving hand to the back of your head and press in that direction also about an inch and release forward. Next, press sideways into your hand being sure that you tilt your head in a side bend so that your chin moves opposite the direction that the top of your head moves. It's fine to just use one hand, but if you want to sense more clearly, use both hands. Repeat in the other direction. When you use rotation, have your hand lower on your face so that the heel of the hand is closer to your jaw. This will engage the sternocleidomastoid muscles more fully; the muscles that connect to the deeper fascial layers.

If you feel confident in your sensing abilities and can control of the rate and gentleness of the exercise, you can begin to stack the articulations. You would combine the motions of rotation and side-bending with flexion or extension, finding the positions of the least resistance and hold it for a few seconds until you feel something soften and let go. You're still moving only an inch in each direction. After feeling a release in the direction of ease, repeat the process using directions of tension, but just stack one at a time. Another helpful if not revealing movement would be to slowly turn your head in one direction while slowly moving your eyes in the opposite direction. The activation of the eyes could recruit and awaken many areas of the brain that may help reset the neck and eye muscles at the same time, while also tying into the shoulders and fascial chains that may be woven into that particular web of tension. Since the eyes are involved in most every action during waking hours, there's a good chance they may be included in the pattern, particularly if time is spent at a computer or doing paper work.

Softening the neck/shoulder junction
There are over 35 muscles in the neck, many of which have attachments in the shoulders. In addition, there are fascial interactions that connect the arms, the spine, the face, and chest to the head. The good thing about that is that we can do movements involving the extremities that result in releasing areas of the head and neck. The other side, of course, is that you'll need to be mindful of how you use your arms throughout the day while healing, because they will be pulling on the neck and head. In these exercises the degree of motion will be greater than those earlier mini- movements, according to tolerance. If you feel comfortable with it, try one action first before combining them. Place a hand on top of your shoulder and press up into your hand toward your ear. Then slowly release the upper trapezius muscle, allowing it to lengthen all the way. Try different hand positions, one at the outermost edge of the shoulder to allow the muscle the most space to move freely, and another with your hands on top of the trapezius so you can sense it as it softens.

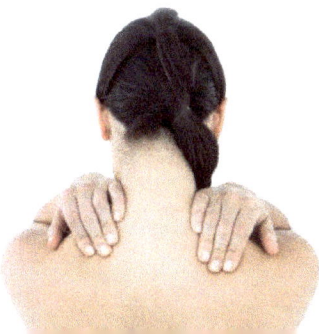

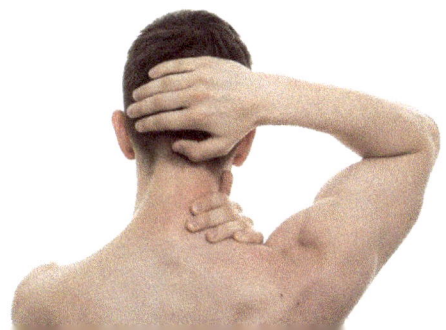

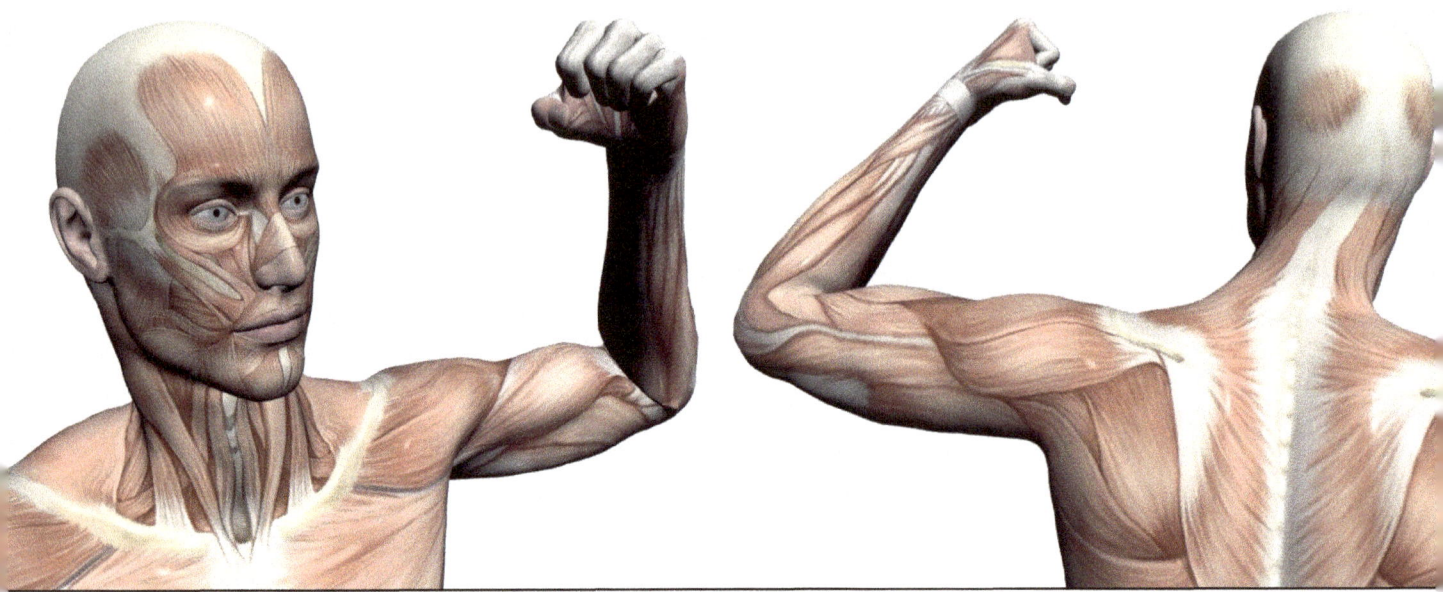

Afterwards you can add the movement of your head going backwards as your shoulder goes up. You should feel the contraction of the neck and shoulder as you resist the pressure of your head with your hands. You'll activate more of the traps if your hand is on the top of the shoulder joint at the head of the humerus where it meets the acromion-clavicular joint. At the height of the contraction, gradually release the muscles and let them lengthen into flexion with your neck, and depression of your shoulder. In other words, you're not pressing them down, but first resisting the elevation and extension, then following the release down towards your feet in the other direction so that the muscles lengthen all the way.

Remember that aerobic exercise is just as important as these more gentle, specific, reeducating movements, because it sends increased levels of blood and oxygen which helps it to be nourished and cleansed, releases inflammation and stress chemistry, and opens soft tissue and organ systems facilitating reset. Balance exercises can engage areas of the brain brought down by brain injury, improving memory, spatial cognition. They effectively activate the cerebellum which coordinates motor activities governing balance, precision, coordination, force, trajectory, and timing. Since the cerebellum interacts with so many other areas of the brain and regulates the information stream in both directions, it is essential to healthy brain function and head trauma recovery. Try several different ways to challenge and re-establish balance, both with eyes open and eyes closed. Be safe though, and hold onto something if you need to. Don't stand near sharp objects.

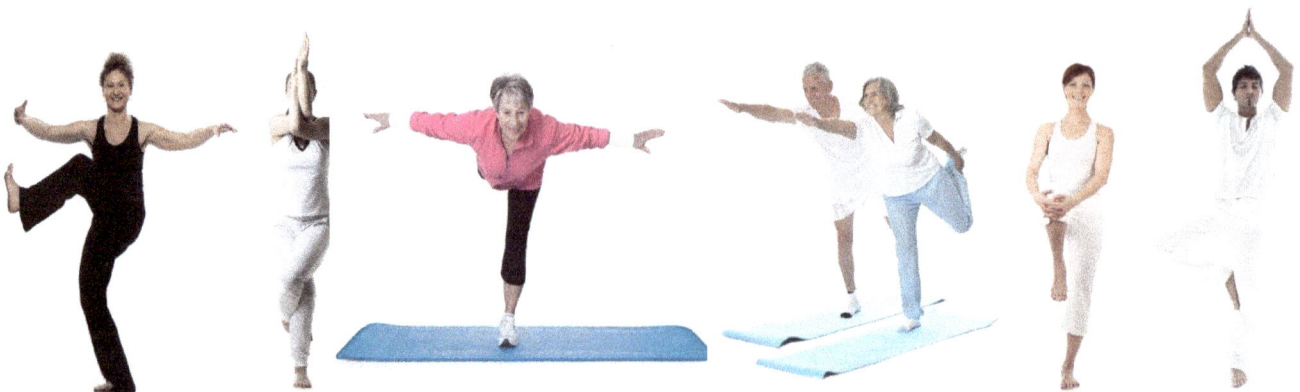

These are easy to do on your own, but it might be helpful to receive guidance initially from a movement coach or physical therapist who can recommend the exercises that will suit you best. Exercise in general improves cognitive function while slowing down volume loss in the hippocampus and frontal lobes. (Rogge, et al, *"Balance training improves memory and spatial cognition in healthy adults"*, Scientific Reports, 2017) Dance can also improve many cognitive and sensory-motor skills when someone is learning new sequences over a period of time. The same results are not found when repeating dance moves that one already knows.

I'll re-emphasize the message now that there are different aspects of a fall, accident, or head trauma that cause brain injury that may need to be treated separately. Diet and supplements will cover one aspect; exercise and reeducation movements serve another. Activities or exercises for the senses, for sensory-motor integration, aphasia, balance, spatial integration, memory, muscle tightness, coordination, and emotional areas – although there may be some overlap – could need to be addressed, assessed, and treated individually. Some of the cognitive issues could correct with time as the brain heals, and some may need additional nutrition or retraining.

I personally found that the sensitivity in the eyes was among the most lasting symptoms, possibly because the eyes tie into so many areas of the brain they are so vulnerable to fatigue. It helps tremendously to work on them directly, or to feel into settling the ascending pathways via the thalamus or wherever you notice the buzz. The digital age isn't as easy on the eyes (or ears) as the analog system. The areas where prior adhesions from early surgeries left a lasting distortion of the tissue field, like the throat and abdomen are also susceptible to creating binding issues preventing the force of subsequent accidents from passing through easily. Scar tissue is also a good place to look when you're considering where residuals are getting hung up. Even the laparoscopic tubal ligation surgery I had continued to challenge the capacity of that hip joint to transmit forces accurately or effectively and likely still creates some error messages for the brain.

That being said, I hope the point was brought home that there are so many remedies that can be sought with manual therapy professionals, and through becoming more awakened and aware in your own system, that the majority if not all of your health can be restored even after a series of serious injuries. The other side of the looking glass means that now you are seeing and sensing your body from within its own sensory mechanisms rather than through the mirror. You're on the other side of your skin, looking in. From this perspective is where the magic happens. Consciousness is a huge part of the recovery process and a support for all other areas of healing. That awareness will effectively guide you in the optimal direction for your unique return to well-being.

The Kingpin epiphany

Bowling has truly been a door to greater insight into the unresolved issues in my throat. Attempting to use a slightly heavier ball (to knock down more pins) than felt comfortable was revealing. The extra weight of the ball pulled just enough up through my arm, neck, spine, and head to create an exacerbation of symptoms. It wound up replicating in a softer way, many of the earlier symptoms of several of the worst incidents. I was eager to get to the bottom of the issue and began to research a little further. What I found was the kingpin to all of the remaining symptoms, similar to the deep cervical fascia.

The cervical fascia, as described earlier, is connected to several structures, some of which are blood vessels and nerves. A significant intersection that plays into many of these structures that throw injury symptoms into a loop is the second cervical vertebrae. It was recently discussed how it relates to the eyes and can be a place to address for headaches as well as eye strain. There is also a nerve plexus there that fans up the back of the head, around the front of the neck and up the face.

A concussion will easily provoke a pain syndrome involving this segment and the one below. They reach every place that the lingering pain expresses itself in my case. These nerves are known to produce migraines, neuralgia, headaches behind the eyes, global tension and pain that are so intense and intractable that nerve blocks are often used to contain them. Irritation of the neck can be a trigger, or the almighty stress factor. In my case, wearing sunglasses or reading glasses that were too heavy could also start the ball rolling. The network is so widespread and capable of producing such diffuse pain patterns that they'd be difficult to allow the main instigator to be identified so it could be treated; like finding a needle in a haystack.

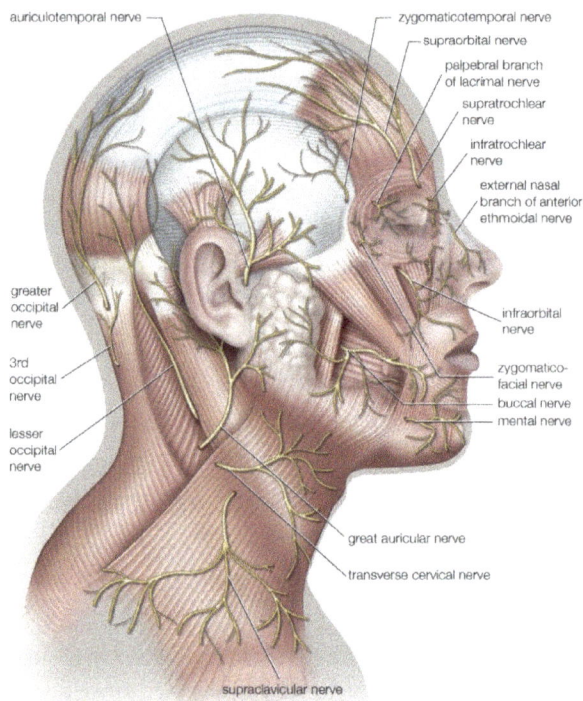

Cutaneous nerves of head and neck

auriculotemporal nerve
greater occipital nerve
3rd occipital nerve
lesser occipital nerve
zygomaticotemporal nerve
supraorbital nerve
palpebral branch of lacrimal nerve
supratrochlear nerve
intratrochlear nerve
external nasal branch of anterior ethmoidal nerve
infraorbital nerve
zygomatico-facial nerve
buccal nerve
mental nerve
great auricular nerve
transverse cervical nerve
supraclavicular nerve

If you're off the mark with this type of pain, it could easily become aggravated and get worse, even if you're being gentle. For example, pulling the ears straight out to the side instead of downward if you're in this syndrome could make it worse. I learned to leave the area alone because I'd made it worse so many times while experimenting with different approaches. Since the supraclavicular nerves fan out across the clavicle, carrying a shoulder strap purse, or backpack could set it off, or make it more tender. I discovered that my first and second ribs were a little out of place and being compressed by the lats, teres, and serratus anterior superior.

These are areas prone to becoming sensitized and registering various pressures or sensations as being painful. For some reason, the sternoclavicular and superior anterior serratus area are often tender in women, possibly due to the heavy lifting we often do with a physique that is not ideally equipped to handle it easily. There are blood vessels, lymph ducts, small ligaments, cervical muscle insertions, bony attachments, meridians and glands, in addition to several nerve fibers that all intersect in or near this thoracic inlet area. I found relief by adjusting the ribs, and the supraclavicular nerve immediately settled down. Consider the efficacy of treating soft tissue through bone, including intraosseous methods.

Only certain substances are effective for the type of nerve pain that comes from injury trauma, and there's no guarantee that it will continue to work, so it's best if at all possible to work with natural remedies and natural analgesics. In my case, Traumeel or even tiger balm could help to dampen some of the tenderness sensation around the clavicle and neck, and stimulating the lymphatic and interstitial fluids toward the thoracic inlet and down the neck settled the irritation measurably. Whatever you find that helps nerve irritation, consider rotating the methods so that the system doesn't adapt to it. Ice usually helps also, but once you get to the root of it – in this case a subluxation caused by muscle tension – it should be easily resolved.

Veins and nerves of the neck

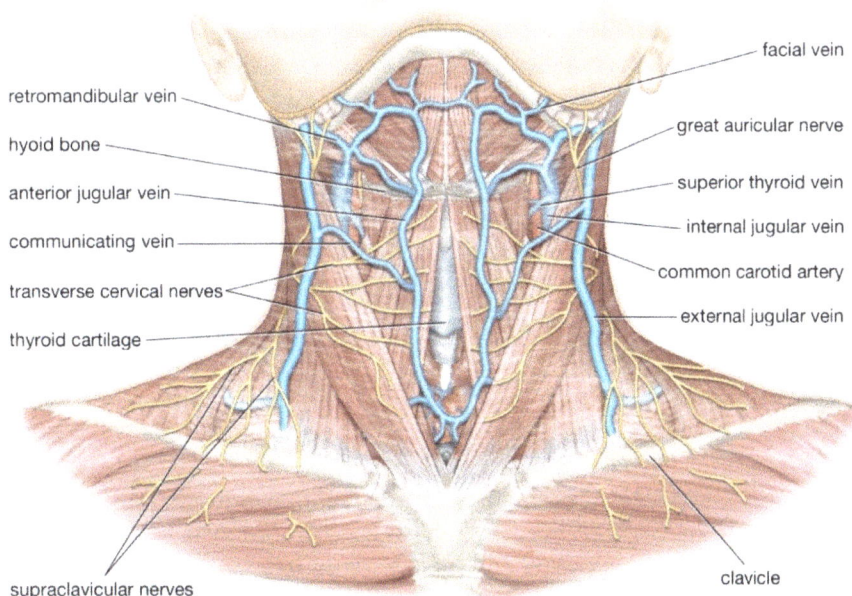

facial vein
retromandibular vein
great auricular nerve
hyoid bone
superior thyroid vein
anterior jugular vein
internal jugular vein
communicating vein
common carotid artery
transverse cervical nerves
external jugular vein
thyroid cartilage
supraclavicular nerves
clavicle

It made sense to address the cervical plexus along with the branches that were flaring up, so I began to track C2, C3 and the brachial plexus to see what that unveiled. There's almost always something in the suboccipital area or at the occiput itself that's paired with the brachial plexus. I decided to use topical analgesics and ice on the plexuses including an Ayurvedic cream all along the transverse cervical nerve. This was the 'collar' I'd so often mentioned over the years to my osteopath that felt unwell and that I was afraid to have anyone touch. Finally I had a name and a location to the trigger. As usual, the initial reaction by contacting this network intensified the pain which was hiding underneath the surface sensations into the deeper fascial layers reflecting in trigger points or subcutaneous nerve pain. This time I'm diving in.

The Kingpin's web of many tails

I settled into a deeper fluid tide and listened. The first 'pull' that the field pointed to as being related was on the frontal side of the skull near the falx cerebri. This was another sensitive trigger starting near the bridge of the nose where a branch of the external carotid artery terminates and Bladder 1 and 2 begin. The entire meridian, all the way down the back, hip and leg, and around the lateral epicondyle of the ankle to the baby toe was tender. I then remembered that my scalp had been tender as long as I could remember, since my mother tried to comb my hair as a small child. Those falls and stitches had an unrecognizable after-effect and set the stage for the present-day syndrome. Approaching the sensitivity through the meridian near the glabella until that area of the eye socket was no longer sore, I worked the carotid artery and the aorta until they felt freer.

My thinking was that freeing the blood and lymph vessels adjacent to the nerves would support the clearing of inflammatory chemistry while the fascia was being opened around them. I then initiated movements that included the neck, shoulder, hips, spine and ankles until nothing was pulling on my neck. I repeated the movements with my tongue out, feeling for maximum tension, working my way through the combined motion of the joints until my tongue and neck felt free more and more deeply. I hadn't found a direct approach that didn't exacerbate, and even though the freedom was greater as was the functions enhanced, the fire still rose up.

I began breathing freer immediately after the deep fascia around my trachea was released, and a chain reaction of ease spread through my system. I slept more deeply than I had in a very long time. The next day the nerves were on fire again. Tension unwinding into inflammation is common in my system. I decided to be specific with where my attempts to cool it down would be. After icing the transverse cervical nerve on the neck, I iced the greater occipital nerve just a bit, then went for the branches that were nearest the subclavian artery. That spot was more tender than all the rest. I then placed the ice on C2 which helped a lot. This whole process took about 15 minutes. After the icing I applied

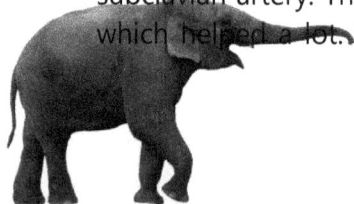

homeopathic ointment to the sternoclavicular joint and along the back of the sternocleidomastoid muscle where the transverse cervical nerve begins its path toward the front of the neck.

I took serrapeptase again before going to bed and had another wonderful night's sleep. In the morning I once again stimulated and augmented the cranial rhythm, which was sluggish at the sacrum; but soon sent soothing waves through my system. I'm still banking on the theory that using the fluid systems to heal the nervous system is the way to go, now that the kingpin has been identified. If it were any other time I'd be satisfied with the results and continue with my daily life knowing that nothing else was needed and move on. This time I'm going to use an essential oil blend that targets nerve irritation and continue to apply it for several days to these key areas to see if it can really heal it so that it doesn't flare again. The oil blend I made for nerve pain included chamomile, ginger, black pepper, lavender, frankincense and lemon balm in a base of jojoba and apricot oils.

The contemplation the following morning took me to C2 and the eyes, particularly the left eye where there'd been an astigmatism since childhood. Self-sensing took my awareness into and through the optic chiasm to the visual geniculate bodies, resting a hand on the posterior thalamus which was pretty buzzy. Sensing there with one hand while the fingers of the other hand wrapped around the body of the left eye spread a global release across the base of the brain, the sub-occipital soft tissue, and down my right hip and leg. To this day my eyes are much less sensitive to light, even in broad daylight. This was a change that was 40 years in the making. This may have been possible due to the releases already made on the deep cervical fascia and cervical plexus extensions; it's a little perplexing.

When I palpated the right hip, there was very little action throughout the iliac artery, but particularly the internal branch. In waiting for that section of the artery to engorge and elongate, a generalized release began to happen all around the greater trochanter on that side, revealing several areas of 'velcro'-like skin that felt similar to that on the neck and collar bone which lit up via the cutaneous nerves. When I applied skin rolling to that area, it took me to the old tubal ligation scar and all the stretch marks under my navel that couldn't be seen when I was pregnant. The pelvic diaphragm was now mirroring the thoracic diaphragm with the intensity of cutaneous nerve irritation.

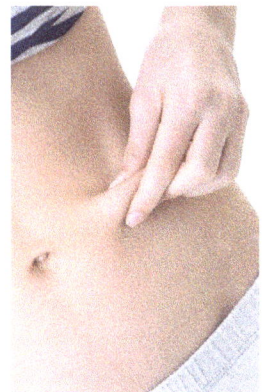

The area near the tubal ligation scar had remained somewhat tender and irritated through the years, often referring into the iliopsoas area and capturing the cecum. In releasing the internal iliac artery, the carotid artery began to feel relieved as did the surrounding tissue and adjacent nerve supply. As helpful as the perfusion of the arteries was, peeling them out of the fascia was the lynch pin. Both areas had been subject to some strain during bowling, as I've often felt a catch in the right hip at the release of the ball. As described in the reports on how the extra-cellular matrix functions, adhesions anywhere in the web can alter the flow of information and create numerous inaccuracies going to and from the brain.

In my case there were many tails that could pull the elephant back into an episode, many of which were near old scar tissue. I'm eager to see how this pans out after monitoring these areas for the subcutaneous and cutaneous sticky spots. This is a factor that also would not be solved by massage, chiropractic, exercise, or t'ai chi-like movements. These burning, tender, restricted layers of the matrix would have to be rolled out, or gently separated by a skilled rolfer or myofascial release practitioner. I can see how something like fibromyalgia could develop from these systems remaining unaddressed, or even develop into an auto-immune issue.

Throughout the years I'd always taken serrapeptase and stopped there once the pain subsided beneath the threshold again and went on with my life. I just didn't want to poke the bear, but being tenacious has really paid off as it only took a few days for the pain to subside and deeper healing to follow. The biggest boon is that now the diffuse pain pattern is demystified and I'll know what to address should it rise again. Even the dry mouth that accompanied the head injury for months was triggered by this process and released in the same day using the related nerve pathways to the parotid and sublingual glands.

I believe I learned from yesterday's pain patterns. Inflammation is the body's correct response to what it perceives as injury, just like a fever tries to burn through a virus or infection. It was too much for the system to process when I included all the layers together – arteries, nerves, fascia, and fluids – while engaging the layers in a global movement. Sometimes less is more. This morning I just focused on the subcutaneous nerves around the right hip and pelvic bowl. I just held the most sensitive spots, but this time it wasn't where a nerve enters soft tissue, it was where the nerve entered the bone. The periosteum of the ASIS, the iliac crest, greater trochanter, and tibia were lit up. I could feel that working this way either released areas above and below, or triggered them. Either way was good information.

The perfusion of the iliac and femoral artery greatly increased, which softened and opened the surrounding fascia and muscle groups. I began including inversion and eversion of the right ankle – the one that had been sprained five times – because it was clearly involved and quite painful. A rash had developed (a couple years ago) over the

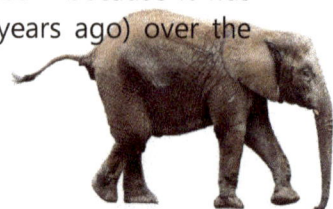

thickest adhesions and the subtalar joint was burning. I'd also torn ligaments on this foot during martial arts, and was beginning to connect the dots between adhesions in the foot and the hip from kicking. Cross-fibering those adhesions enabled that stubborn rash to finally begin to dissipate and regroup into normal skin again. It's also beginning to seem like calming the exacerbation through the arteries is the most readily accepted by my body.

The sural nerve just beneath the lateral epicondyle (ankle bone) was definitely the nerve that was sending pain up the chain. Since it is a branch of the sciatic nerve, it is easily able to influence the leg and hip. After opening the fascia and vessels around the right hip and working the right ankle in connection just a bit, I again fell into a deep sleep. Not having the type of subliminal nerve irritation that disrupts sleep patterns would be a huge bonus to this exploration. Everything felt better in the morning and the skin around my pelvis remained supple and had lost that burning, Velcro stickiness. This line from the neck to the pelvis was carved out by the whiplash many years ago, but had been enlivened by the strikes to the top of the head. Nonetheless, starting at the feet or center of gravity didn't trigger the thoracic diaphragm, cervical or cranial area, but working in those pelvic areas could trigger everything inferior to them.

Perhaps I shouldn't have been surprised, but the third day the pain diminished almost entirely after eating a piece of lamb. Somehow the nutrients in red meat are extremely helpful for my nervous system and what it needs to heal. A few additional discoveries happened that day when feeling into the precise areas of lingering tenderness. One of the spots was near the back of the mastoid bone in the groove where the attachment to the digastric muscle sits. When I followed it over to the hyoid bone, I could see that the origin was also sore, as well as the cricothyroid and sternohyoid muscles. It's possible that singing in ranges that are too high for my voice hasn't been helpful for this syndrome, but I'm remembering now that a vocal coach had a technique to stick out your tongue and hold it with your fingers while singing the scales. This exercise may be needed at least until it fully heals.

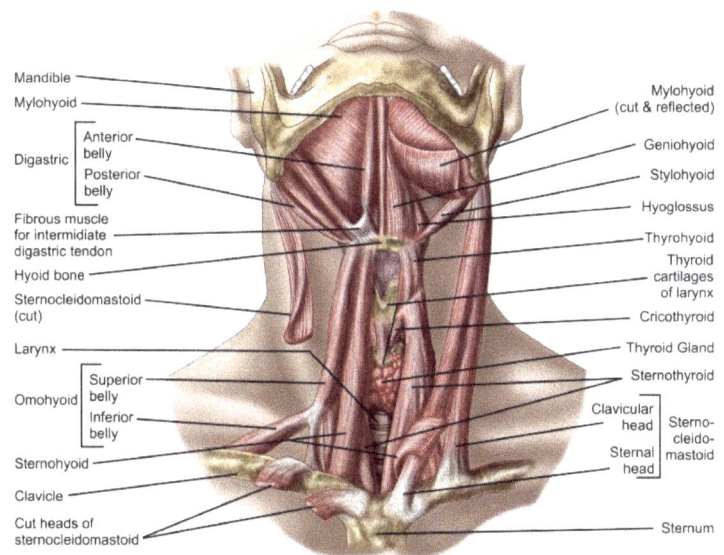

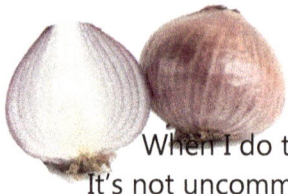

When I do that now I can feel it pulling to the left although the burning is on the right. It's not uncommon for the tender side to be opposite the tight one. The burning tightness is deep, while the tender pain registers in the superficial nerves. The recurrent laryngeal nerve was quite hot, as was the adjacent terminal junction at the insertion of the anterior scalenes and sternohyoid insertion. The fascia running along the midline from the sling that supports the hyoid bone up through to the mental edge of the chin was all hot. Releasing this piece of the anterior cervical fascia ligament did wonders for the sub-occipital area and seemed to release an 'antsy' agitation in my system that could have manifested as ADD.

It's pretty amazing how the adaptations and subliminal tensions can exist under the radar for so long, all the while being the substrate for that condition called 'chronic'. It can also be the substrate for low-grade inflammation and poor sleep that can have significant health implications in the long run. By the third day of my self-treating explorations I could read more easily in dim light and was receiving the sunlight even better. I began tracking the sore spots with more pressure, and instead of irritated nerves and arteries, found very tight muscles that likely have been that way for most of my life. One area was that of the auricularis group that flanks the ear on all sides and lead quite naturally into the temporalis muscle that felt like stone. I'm pretty sure the braces at age 14 contributed to this tension, as they didn't allow for the natural cranial motion for a couple of years.

I'm gathering up all of these tails, but my guess now is that the mama elephant for the thoracic diaphragm is C2 and the brachial plexus. All the baby tails are tied to her and the area to the right of C7 is tight and sore. The hip and ankle seemed tertiary, while the throat and glabella seem primary and secondary to the flare-ups. My first falls down the stairs as a child were onto my face, and if nothing else had happened, they most likely could have been absorbed without notice. Now, the sensitized glabella responds amazingly well to clearing the bladder meridian as well as using cranial compress-decompress methods that include the facial bones.

The serratus anterior were probably still holding on from the thousands of push-ups I did decades ago, complicated by the phrenic nerve activation that ties into the greater occipital nerve, C2, and the intercostal nerves, each of which were on hyper mode from the head injuries. Addressing the phrenic and vagus nerves near the diaphragm released the persistent, recent bout of nausea, and adjusting the ribs was able to help the clavicle quite a bit. The transverse cervical nerve and cervical fascia are settling down and my neck muscles in general feel pliant and soft. Applying the essential oil I made laterally, first following, then opposing rotation, seemed to open the layers of cervical fascia and made my neck feel brand new.

After addressing the cricothyroid muscles around the larynx and the auricular muscles surrounding the right ear, I could hear a new resonance in my head while singing and harmonies were easier to find. There's more to be done with the auricularis group, as they appear to be in relationship to the masseter, temporalis and pterygoids. Even so, my breathing is easier and more spacious, and my spine released down to the tailbone as it does with the jaw work. These discoveries will likely not be a 'one and done' situation, but require an ongoing monitoring and movement reeducation for a while to reinforce the changes and make them last.

I certainly won't avoid or subdue pain like that again, and will advise clients to look under that threshold for pain and uncover what well may be setting up a scenario for chronic, low grade inflammation that could lead to other more uncomfortable conditions in the future. During the exacerbation of symptoms in this exploration, many cognitive symptoms returned, as though the inflammation and reorganization of fascia over nerves and vessels threw my brain into confusion, even though I was sleeping well and hydrating.

It took about a week for that aspect to resolve, supported by a little gotu kola more than fish or anything else. There's still additional improvement to be had with a few cranial and occipital nerves, but I already feel better than I have in many years. Mind you, I was already feeling 80% recovered, but now feel I'm approaching 90% and intending to nourish heal the CNS so it's not so sensitized and triggerable. Finding ways to protect, nourish and strengthen the glial cells which can in turn repair and nourish the nerve cells feels like a good goal. I think I'll increase the essential fatty acids and see where that goes.

Epiphany within the epiphany

I was about to complete this book and then something remarkable happened. I wondered what wanted to surface next. There was a bit of tinnitus and a lot of buzz that woke me up this morning, so I settled into a cranial tide and followed the pulls, many of which were in the head. The scar tissue near the right hip was also zinging, and appeared to be related. I remembered a process in a couple of classes that had an energetic component whereby lines of energy in the system could connect and resolve once the connection was addressed. Since the lynch pins were most often near surgeries, I tried to remember what else was going on in my life at the time of the surgeries and the game-changing fall.

Sure enough, there were specific emotional conflicts with family at the time of the surgeries, stitches, the punch in the throat, and the fall. In the case of the nasal surgery when I was five, there was a single traumatic event whereby four hospital interns held me down by all four limbs as I was screaming and kicking until they put the nozzle over my face emitting ether. That drama went into the adhesion. In the case of the braces being

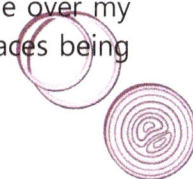

installed - which in those days involved metal bands being glued and hammered into your gums - I was passing out from the pain of it. The dentist put down his instruments, walked out of the room and came back in and said that President Kennedy had just been shot. He grabbed my face with all his stressed-out feelings and said, "I can't do this unless you hold still!" I was limp and almost unconscious and couldn't control my body at that point. Neither I nor my system was able to process the new braces effectively, much less the dentist and the death of our President.

Some of the strands that were still tangling and sensitizing the web were the emotional impressions that had fired and wired at the same time. They were now presenting as the searing pain part of the syndrome that resided in the superficial and subcutaneous nerve fibers. From there that emotional chameleon could slip into fluids, fascia, joints, or wherever the network enlivened. Therein lies that extra spark of unresolved kindling that was ripe for the fire of exacerbation. The symptoms as well as their location could vary and be harder to identify since the memories were from a variety of incidents over a long period of time. It's not like I hadn't addressed these incidents or these emotions before, but they hadn't been linked together in time, physical form, content, energy, and physiology before.

They say that the layers keep peeling off, either to reveal deeper issues, or to reveal deeper levels of the same issue. I also feel that when some of the snags in the fabric unwind, the remaining snags become more apparent. My manual therapy teachers have said that once the body runs out of space it begins to store trauma in the bones. I have to believe that even though so much healing had happened, with the periosteum being as tender as it was in so many different areas, that I was again on the verge of running out of reserves. In the case of these numerous injuries over the years, that cervical kingpin area was the key to it all, along with one other key area: the 'me' area of the brain that revealed itself as part of the fabric this morning. From the organizing principle of the fluid tide, the old scars were lighting up in the tissue, nerves, and brain simultaneously.

The right parietal region, where researchers found that the 'experiencing ego or entity' resides neurologically, was now ablaze. This region where the brain 'you' lives has captured those traumas and is holding them in trust. It's different than a stored memory in the hippocampus; it's more like a CNS gestalt of who you are. There is a Zero Balancing Bodywork method that scans and connects to energetic restrictions from the shoulders, whereas in Barral's Manual Thermal Evaluation method the scan and connection happens from the right parietal area of the brain. His approach includes a feedback aspect rather than just the feedforward. In this way the brain 'you' is able to receive updated information from the old wounds and reorganize accordingly. For some reason, part of the discharge included a lot of coughing and a few sneezes as these impressions were being dislodged.

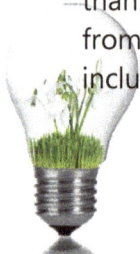

In any case, I went to the entry and exit meridian points for the lungs, large intestines, bladder, gall bladder, and kidney to support the energetic releases. Those points were tender, except for the kidney entry point. As the energy along the kidney meridian dissipated, so did a great deal of the sensitivity along the periosteum of the tibia, clavicle, sternum, and iliac crest. I think I'll also need to visit the cervical plexus, as one of my teachers mentioned that they function as gatekeepers to block trauma from reaching the brain, so that could be another reason why they're part of the kingpin. Touching in at the neck, the pull was posterior and inferior to the sacrum. That will be my next pairing along with the cerebellum, but now will let the system rest and integrate.

"As the most fundamental of all connective tissues, bone serves a scaffolding function in the formation and the shape of the organization. Bones are basic in the physical expression of the life force, macroscopically and microscopically. The artistry of dance and the dance of biochemistry represent two ends of the spectrum of the life force manifested in bone."(R. Paul Lee, DO, Interface, Mechanisms of Spirit in Osteopathy, 2005)

Another Aha!

I thought the last epiphany would be the last Aha! for this text, but most likely others pieces of the puzzle will continue to reveal themselves as the quest for 100% healing continues. The one that came this morning was whether or not the intraosseous compression of the cranial bones had been addressed in a specific way. There had certainly been adequate mobilization of the bones and fluids therapeutically, and a few general compress/decompress methods had been applied all over my skull, but I wasn't thinking of the periosteum and the internal cancellous portion of the flat bones. Barral had mentioned in class that trauma can land in the bones, and when the bone itself receives a direct hit, it now seems logical that a portion of the trauma could settle inside of the bony matrix.

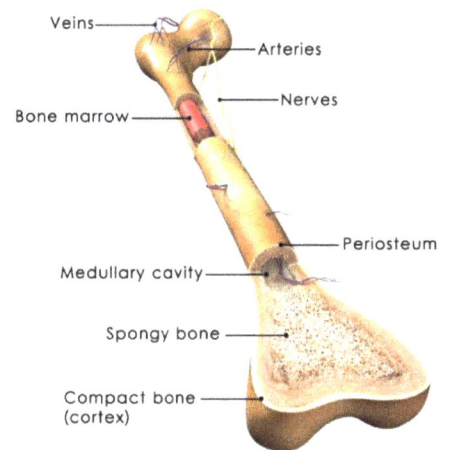

The main difference between this focus and that of the compress/decompress approach is that the latter does an awesome job of allowing the dural and sub-dural tissues to reorganize, whereas this intent is on the interior of the bones. I was imagining the layer where the nerves and blood vessels enter the compact bone layer, but also the deeper spongy layer of the marrow where more significant functions occur. In the case of flat bones, making new blood cells is their main role but in long bones there are many regulatory support functions. There is a bone remodeling process that happens in

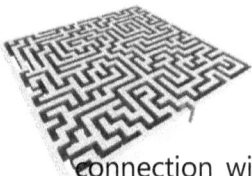

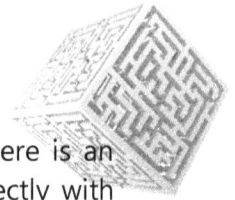

connection with the kidneys, thyroid and nervous system in the bones, and there is an endocrine function related to insulin sensitivity whereby the bones interact directly with the pancreas.

Bones have an immune system, acting as first responders for inflammation. They store energy and absorb toxins, they help maintain the acid/alkaline balance in the body, and the hormone osteocalcin plays a role in the cortex whereby mood and cognitive functions have been shown to be affected. (Oury, Khrimian, et al, *"Maternal and Offspring Pools of Osteocalcin Influence Brain Development and Functions"*, Cell, Sept. 2018). In fact, some dementia patients have been observed to have low levels of osteocalcin, which research shows has a direct relationship with the hippocampus in addition to being able to affect states of anxiety and depression. (Karsenty et al, *"Bone Hormone Influences Brain Development and Cognition,"* Columbia University Medical Center Newsroom, 2013) We've talked more about overlapping structures than overlapping functions so far, but a structure and its function are inseparable.

There are many forms of communication and types of pathways that carry information from cell to cell within and between structures, and in this instance, whatever system was being used by the flat bones, the shift was instantaneous among nearly all of them. The flat bones include the cranial bones, the pelvis, sternum, vomer, ribs, lacrimal bones (medial part of eye socket), scapula, and nasal bone – all of which have been tender. The skin over the ilium and sternum have been much less tender, as has the tissue over the clavicle since it was rolled out and had the essential oil blend applied. After supporting the release of the intraosseous stress in the bones of the skull, not only do all of the flat bones and the joints that attach to them feel normal again, but the area of the tibia that chronically felt like shin splints recently has also normalized. Of course nothing in life is static, and I don't imagine that this is a permanent fix, but a remarkable revelation full of possibilities for how to approach this type of imbalance.

I never would have looked at the tapestry of bone as having a cross-talk of pain, and I'm excited to see if the irregular bones will also respond if I explore further. So far, my posture was effortlessly erect immediately after this self-treatment session, and both shoulders gained that extra 5% in their range of motion, each of which had a slight residual restriction from their prior adhesive capsulitis. Surprisingly, the biggest changes happened after working with the frontal bone, particularly in the spots where there'd been stitches.

I became curious about the source of inflammatory chemistry and decided to take advantage of the next time the 'fire' of irritation began in the residual areas of the neck and cranial base, which hadn't entirely receded. I felt into the fire as an element from the

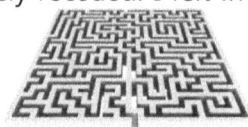

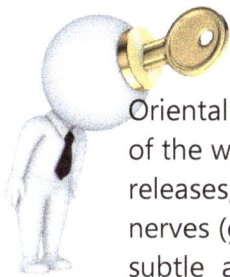

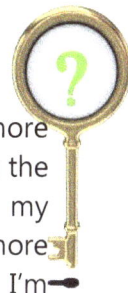

Oriental Medicine perspective and wondered if tuning in to the kidneys would bring more of the water element to bear. That helped some, but when I began to cough again with the releases, I checked into the element of air. As space opened out around the 'fire' in my nerves (greater occipital and transverse cutaneous), it led me to the element of ether, more subtle and more still than breath. Then the nerves really began to calm down. I'm interpreting ether as that state that may arise in meditation, although there is a type of void that opens up after inhaling before exhaling that also sets the stage for a fulcrum in the system to reorganize and settle down. I often hold my breath while working on clients because there's more receptivity and enhanced listening ability in the quietness of it.

Various organs (liver, intestines, heart, spleen, lungs) were stimulated in the process of this inquiry, revealing their association with the elemental nature and frequencies of our systems. Balance in the elements is just as important as balance in the musculo-skeletal structures and functions. The healing process proved to be more of a holistic one than I could have imagined. Truly every system and layer thereof had been affected and attempting to hold its own over the years. Timing is key in choosing which layer to approach at which phase of the process, and it may be unique to each person. Today was the correct time to open and also balance the flow of energy, whereas when the fire's blazing, it's like pouring gasoline on the fire.

Approaching your system with fresh curiosity and listening each time is going to be very helpful, just like a surfer doesn't go in the water without knowing what the conditions are each time. The types of releases that came with these most recent explorations can be helpful even if you haven't had concussions or brain injuries. Sticky, compressed places can arise from surgeries or even daily wear and tear if not seen for periodic maintenance. As a martial artist, dancer, and athlete, I can attest that in middle age the impacts of all those activities come knocking on the door of your reserves and resiliency. I wish I'd known then what I know now, but am grateful now to have been able to unravel the build-up in time. To support the recent openings I increased a few supplements. I can feel a difference already in a few days of taking the Essential Fatty Acids (Omega-3, DHA & EPA) and B-Complex more often. Oddly, I'm much less hungry, as if part of my appetite was geared toward feeding my struggling brain.

The crux of the Kingpin

There may be another layer that needs attention. Many nights there have appeared to be light particles hitting my body in a specific way, and at times I stayed awake and looked into it further. I knew they bounced up against areas of tension repeatedly, like they were pointing out areas that they couldn't pass through, and I knew that holding the cell phone to my head earlier in the day had created a greater disturbance in how they behaved. On these nights I generally have to work a bit more to harmonize the effects on

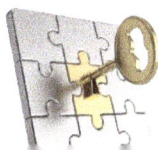

my brain. Since the sound carrying those EMF's goes in through the ears, I can usually calm and balance the frequencies by placing my fingertips in my ears, listening for that void state, which Bhagwan would call the 'sound of one hand clapping', and waiting for the discharge to happen.

This time I got more interested in what was happening in the tissue fields since I now am more aware of which fascia connects the ears to the nose and throat - the area of the kingpin. The temporal bones were moving just fine, but were not in sync, and as usual, one ear canal was tighter and smaller than the other. When I focused on that fact with attention to the deeper fascia behind the canal, adjustments began to occur that revealed the residual shearing and torsion in the brain tissue. Contacting that distortion in a physical way opened the neurophysiology of it and the irritation of the plexus at C2, the greater occipital, transverse cervical, facial, trigeminal, andl glossopharyngeal nerves. I now could see in real time the cause of the hemiplegic migraines and trigeminal neuralgia after the game-changer.

The area of the auricularis muscles as well as the cricothyroid and sternohyoid muscles lit up. On the other end, the pelvic bowl, cauda equina area, and calves relaxed and opened more and more. Now it seems that the intracranial distortions sent the firestorm throughout the central nervous system, the peripheral and subcutaneous nerves including those that innervate layers of fascia and periosteum. The more that layer released, the more the point of impact on the occiput lit up. When I looked to the element of ether to calm the storm, the light particles in the room stimulated my curiosity about biphotons. Could they be yet another tail of the elephant; another piece of the puzzle? Biophotons both hold memory and transmit information between cells. Fritz Popp has been researching biophotons for over four decades and find that, *"the biophotons emitted from our cells are highly coherent energy that may be responsible for the operation of our biological systems."* (*Biophoton: The Light in Our Cells*, Dr. Joe Depsez'a Blog", August, 2016)

Popp and Cohen report after observing 200 people, *"biophoton emissions reflect a) the left-right symmetry of the human body, b) biological rhythms, c) disease in terms of broken symmetry between left and right side, and d) light channels in the body which regulate energy and information transfer between different parts."* (Indian Journal of Explorative Biology, May, 2003). Also known as ultraweak photon emissions, biophotons exist within the near-infrared through violet range that lives between 200 and 1300 nanometers, which is faintly within the visible spectrum for the naked eye. Russian scientist Gariaev reports that this form of light has memory that can be absorbed and retained by DNA. Bókkon's theory that biophotons are emitted during visual imagery activity in the brain was confirmed by researchers Dotta, Saroka and Persinger. (Neuroscience Lett, April, 2012)

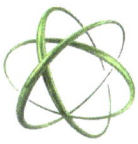

An additional characteristic of biophotons in a rat's brain was described by Kobayashi, Takeda, et. al. as being *"correlated with cerebral energy metabolism and oxidative stress"*. (Neuroscience Research, July 1999) There's more. Neurons in the brain produce biophotons at the estimated potential rate of over a billion per second, which researchers propose could facilitate communication rates that support quantum entanglement. This property, they say, could be the bridge between the human being and consciousness and explain the 'how' behind non-local phenomena. (*"Are There Optical Communication Channels in Our Brains*?" MIT Technology Review, September, 2017; Kumar, Boone, et al, *"Possible existence of optical communication channels in the brain"*, Scientific Reports, November 2016)

There is also support for a *"preferential guidance of light along the axis of white matter tracts of the brain"*. (Hebeda, Menovsky, et al, *"Light propagation in the brain depends on nerve fiber orientation"*, Neurosurgery, October, 1994) Since the white matter is where some of the damage and tearing happens in brain injury, it stands to reason that this conductivity can be disrupted. I had mentioned the conductivity and meridian flow issue several times to practitioners when receiving treatment, but the area is clearly one that has not reached critical mass in a way that it could yet become an area of rehabilitation. In the field of manual therapy, A. T. Still views the field around the body as such: " *The pattern of physcial conformation contains a pattern of charge as well. This holographic pattern of charge in the connective tissues matches a purely energetic pattern of charge, a morphogenetic field."* Paul Lee goes on to say, *"Energy transfers from the spiritual realm to the physical realm and is transduced to metabolic activity as a function of electricity. Still called the electric activity of the body the 'highest known order of force'"*

The meditation practices I had become accustomed to transitioned into contemplation practices partly due to this issue, which I couldn't interpret at the time as being realted to the brain's electrical/light status being disrupted by injury and trauma. I could see that the 'wave had become the particle' in a very real sense. Although there definitely was also an organizing principle with the particle aspect of consciousness or Shakti or active light, it's the wave aspect that is more coherent, more empty, and therefore provides a calmer substrate for the healing to take place in as the Shakti and organizing principle go to work. Is this biophoton field responsible for coherence, or reflecting the status? It appears it could be both, and also carrying the imprint of the injures. That's why I feel that shifting states or using a deeper (cranial) tide in order to bring in new input that doesn't carry that memory would be a worthwhile inquiry while addressing the surface layers.

Healing and integration happen on several different levels and layers, each one bearing its own signature as a way of feeling freer and more balanced. Feeling balanced in the skeletal system is amazing, but very different than feeling integrated through a fluid

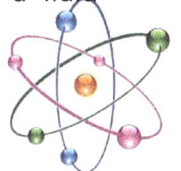

system or tissue field. Each layer may also have a particular key to open the door most easily to that entire web. It may be in the area of lesion, but the it could also be through a less challenging but related structure. Although they are each a web unto itself and definitely interconnected, there hasn't been an instance so far whereby one system was the main integrative factor for all of the others. I'm wondering now if the subtler fields could be the hand that holds all the tails of the elephant and could be the interpenetrating field that resets them all. This field may hold an energetic Akashic record of every incident that, once cleared, would enable changes to last. Not that this field could clear all of the other layers, but when this field is cleared, it could be a factor in the symptoms not returning; like erasing an energetic transmission of the memory.

Meditation is also an incredible organizing force, yet the biophoton system seems to include more of the intelligent, coherent, organizing principle that is reminiscent of the inherent treatment plan in the Biodynamic Cranial model. Whenever I've contemplated these disorganized particles that appear to represent error messages in the bridge between energy/nadis, the nervous system, and the sensory organs and dropped beneath them to a deeper layer of consciousness, the pain vanishes and the tissue fields and nerves feel normal again. It somehow touches back into the space that opened up in India and frees the physical body of even the memory of pain signals. It doesn't erase injury, but switches tracks, adds coherence and such ease at every level, that a deeper sleep can support healing.

I should mention that cell phone or prolonged computer use can distort this field of influence, and can be a triggering force for my system through the eyes or ears, or even the nasal passages if using the speaker phone. By the way, my ear canals are now the same width and there are no pulls when I stick out my tongue. This time I want to see if these particles, whether they are biophotons or not, will release their memory of these accidents so the triggerability will also vanish. My energy level is better now since the residuals aren't occupying the physiology, neurology, meridians, skeletal and tissue fields like they were. An unexpected bonus is that since the 'biophoton' exploration and working at the site of the game-changer, there is highly increased dexterity in my fingers (I'm typing faster now with much greater accuracy.) It could be that the cerebellum or some site responsible for motor execution was served in that session. Somehow the intelligent, organizing principle continues to lead you to the next key to the door of deeper healing.

Contacting the Tide
Once you've shifted perspectives on what the body is and how it functions, it'll be easier to look for motion internally. For as many times over the years that you may have made contact with your body, you weren't expecting organs, fluids, bones, or your brain to be in motion, even though when you think about it, everything rests in a body filled with

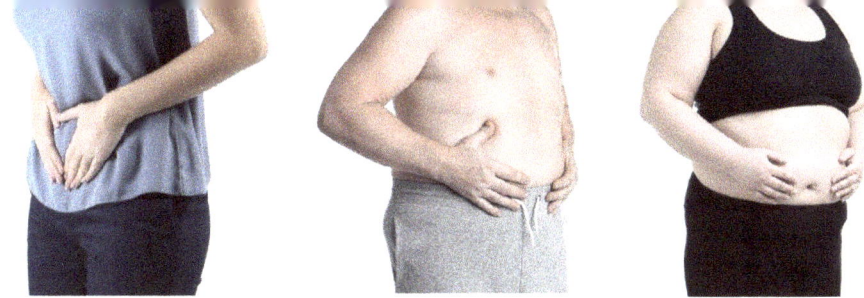

water. Now that you know everything moves, even at the cellular level where countless micro transmissions of information happens, you can more easily palpate for and sense fluid motion in your system. The best area initially to sense movement is in the abdominal area since it's so juicy in there, and as there are several branches of the vagus nerve that terminate in the abdomen, it's a great way to calm the system by a simple, gentle hold. Below the navel is the dan tien, a reservoir of energy often referred to in chi kung that is adjacent to a parasympathetic plexus anterior to the sacrum, so holding the belly below the navel is also a great way to settle the system after an injury.

Sensing at the belly

Softly place your hands – one on top of the other - on your belly, in the area of the umbilicus, and wait until you feel a slight motion, like a boat rocking slightly on top of the water while tied to a dock in a calm Bay. Let your hands move with the underlying movement of the water, taking note of which direction it may be favoring, or if the motion is evenly distributed to the same degree in both directions. Also make note if it's moving in several directions and stay with it, being mindful of any additional sensations that arise, and when the rate, depth, or directions of the movement shift or pause.

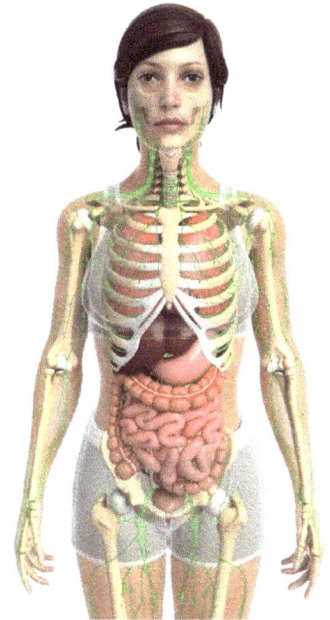

Whatever direction the underlying forces create, go with it and see where it leads or seems to be pointing to. It likely will be leading you to a primary lesion or point of reorganization that needs attention. Then separate your hands with one to the right and the other to the left, or with one above the navel and the other below it, and watch the movement patterns again for a few minutes. The motion generally will fluctuate for a couple of minutes according to whatever forces are present at the time, then fall into a rhythmic pattern either between medial and lateral or between superior and inferior.

If all is well and vital, the rhythmic pattern will express right away but may be mild and gain strength as you provide your presence for a few minutes. With the green lines representing the lymph vessels and nodes, the yellow representing major nerve fibers, and the blue and red

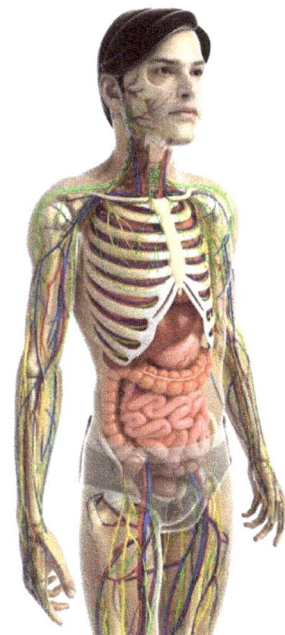

illustrating vein and artery pathways, you can see that there's quite a bit of overlap in these systems and that major intersections happen at the joints where compression can easily occur. These images don't show the infusion of flow into, around, and through the organs, muscles, fascia, skin and bones, but you can imagine how a restriction anywhere can create stagnation in other critical areas. It also helps to imagine what you're touching into when you place your hands over these structures as you rest them in different positions over your abdomen. Listen for any feedback you may be able to receive from a particular organ or system in terms of how bright, light and airy, or dense, stiff, and dull it may feel. Feel the fluids moving around and through these systems and notice when the sensations or feedback changes with the enhancement of Tidal energies and fluids.

Sensing at the sternum

At one point you can move the upper hand a little higher to make gentle contact with the sternum, just in the middle of the ribs and beneath the clavicle. There are several pertinent structures under there that will be helpful in down-regulating your nervous system and relaxing some of the structures that were impacted during an accident. The heart is just behind there surrounded by the pericardium which has links into the buccopharyngeal fascia; the thymus gland sits there, in front of the esophagus which also connects to the deep cervical fascia; and the vagus nerve passes through the lateral aspect of the sternum flanked by the internal thoracic artery and nerve, as well as the aorta, subclavian, and brachiocephalic arteries and major lymph ducts.

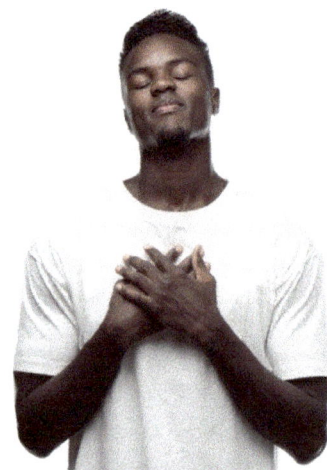

There are also muscle insertions in the first two ribs for the scalenes and sternocleidomastoid muscles, the platysma, along with the sternohyoid muscle that attaches just near the manubrium. It's quite the hub of activity so your contact there will influence many structures and their functions. It's common to feel releases at the occiput, through the neck into the shoulders, in the hips and even down the spine by making contact with this area, which is a vital and pivotal point for whiplash and head injuries. Ideally, you'll also feel an increase in the pulsing of the arteries beneath your hand as the perfusion of blood in them is enhanced by the softening of the vessel walls and surrounding tissues. A little lower beneath the clavicle will be the entry and exit of vessels into the lungs. A shock or trauma has the ability to greatly reduce the movement in these vital structures, which, if it goes on long enough, will begin the express itself in other conditions as the stagnation grows.

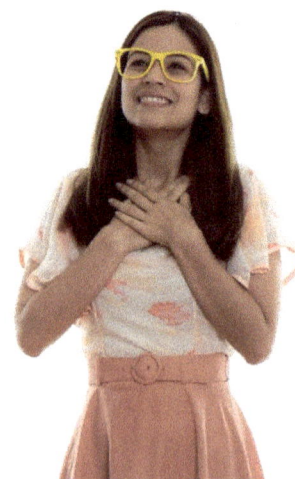

Everyone is not a 'feeling' type and won't be able to pick up tactile or kinesthetic sensations right away, so be patient with the process. Like most things, it gets better with practice and tuning in. In any case, just being present and listening to your belly will generate positive changes toward balance and calm. The more you listen, the more information you'll be able to garner from what the movements are expressing, and from what your system's tendencies are at the time. Even if you never feel things moving and changing from your hands resting on your belly, there will be an ease created that is also helpful for your intestines, bladder, and kidneys as fascial and muscular connections soften.

Sensing at the pelvis

Just beneath the belly is the pelvic girdle which is also a super highway of activity. Placing your hands just on the ASIS – the anterior superior iliac spine - of the pelvis (the most forward bone at the uppermost rim of the pelvic girdle) of the will reveal if one side is lower than the other, or more posterior than the other side, and if there is rhythmic movement happening through the bones along with the soft tissue. There will be a great deal of action here after you've been on a walk, bike ride, or run, as if the body was still in motion although the activity ending while ago. Wait for the bones to stabilize and level out, if they will, then move your hands slightly lower to the inguinal area. If they don't level out on their own, use a few of the global movements described earlier then check the pelvis again and note the changes.

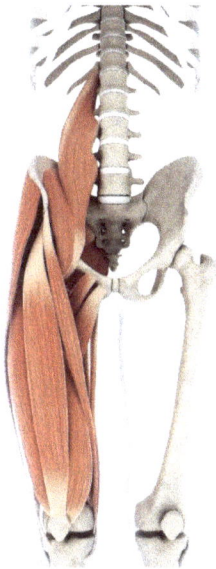

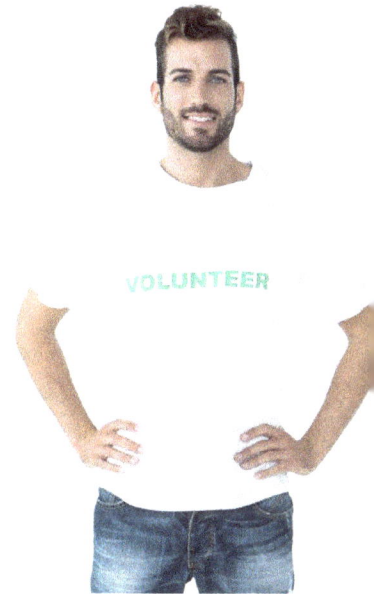

It may reveal that certain imbalances that happen after sitting or standing for long hours, or after sports or hobbies will create imbalances that you can catch and correct right away. If you don't feel easy motion and hearty pulsing of the femoral artery with your hands in the inguinal area, that's also a signal to do some of the lengthening and opening movements to be sure stagnation or restrictions haven't been unwittingly created during the day's activities. Remember that all the nerves and vessels are connected in a seamless network, so restriction in any area has an impact on the other areas. It could be that the flow through the pelvic girdle is light due to restrictions in the aorta or subclavian arteries higher up or vice versa, so it would be a fun ongoing query to compare your activities and accompanying sensations or symptoms to which restrictions appear. It could also work the other way, whereby certain activities or hobbies could open restrictions and stagnation. You can also try placing one hand high on the sternum and the other lower in the belly and see if either pulse, amplitude, or rhythm increases by contacting both simultaneously.

Using meridians to affect the cranium

Another wonderful place to hold and catch the drift of the tide is at the base of the skull, or the occiput. You should notice it swiveling out from the base and back under as the apex (actually at the bottom end) swivels out, in harmony with the motion of the sacrum. It's soothing to hold either one, but test it out for yourself which hand placement brings a sigh of relief and go with that for a while until your body shifts its response with a different area. You can get a sense of whether or not there is movement, whether it feels slight or full, smooth or uneven, racy or slow. Children and pregnant women generally have full, vibrant, even fluid flows, as well as adults after exercising. If it is diminished or uneven, after you hold it for a while, it usually will increase in amplitude and become slower and more even as the system settles and re-regulates itself. It's a very common position we've often used to kick back and relax, so the instincts are there to hold the base of the skull when it's time to let go and chill or regroup.

Not to worry if you don't sense motion. There could be several reasons for that eventuality, many of which would be easily remedied energetically. I'd mentioned earlier that head injuries can cause restrictions in many systems, some of which are energetic. There are several energetic systems, and the meridian system in Chinese medicine is the most well-known one for most households. I've very often opened the cranial bone motion using the bladder and/or gall bladder meridians, as well as the governing vessel, which runs along the falx and straight sinus. Lightly pressing along these pathways two to three times will usually open the bony and fluid flows in the cranium and brain. If there is sensitivity along those pathways, and there may be if there's a restriction, go with lighter pressure and include a few of the points as well as palming the pathways with the heel or edge of your hand. The points would respond better to using just one finger, again pressing lightly three times.

Some teachers in this system have said that experiencing pain (tissue damage notwithstanding) is an indication of blocked energy flow. The points on the forehead can open energy flow, but also allow access by intention to the prefrontal cortex and basal ganglia where mental or emotional stressors may be palpated and settled. If it feels like a row boat in rocky waters, there may be some stress going on. Hold the points and wait for a smooth, steady rhythm to arise. The bladder points near the tear ducts or eyebrow are also areas that are instinctively pressed when the eyes get strained or tired, and even when a headache is starting. It can be a great

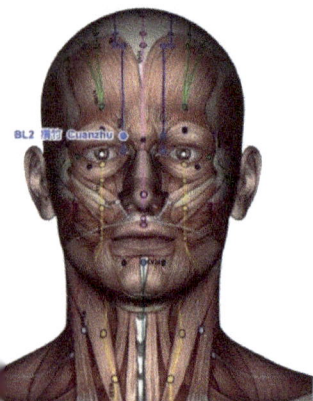

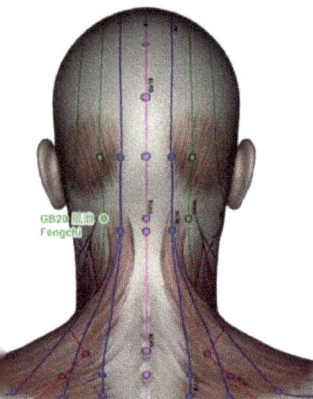

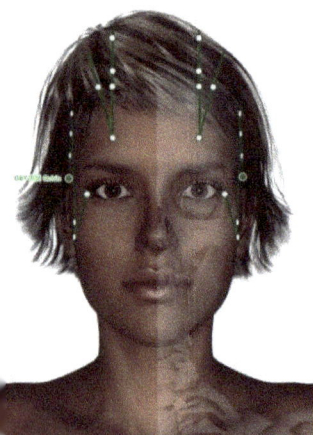

help to lightly stimulate these points for post-concussive symptoms related to eye sensitivity and back tension, as the influence reaches the full length of the meridian. As you become more sensitive, you may be able to discern the change from a buzzy or edgy feel to the energetic flow to a smoother, more easeful, silent presence like a kayak easing through a placid river. Reinforce the energetic and soft tissue openings and with a few of the movement sequences to release the posterior of the body if you want to increase the staying power of the results.

In the beginning you may not feel entirely comfortable or confident in your ability to self-treat in all of these instances, and feel free to visit a manual therapist you have a resonance with to lend a hand or to clarify hand positions for you. As your relationship builds with your system, you'll be more and more effective in getting immediate results, and will also know when to see someone.

Sensing at the cranium

You can begin with one or two hands, but know that your body will always be responding to the position of your hands, and if they aren't completely level, it will change what you feel. If you use two hands you can also compare sides and see if one side is moving more than another, or in a different trajectory, etc. When you use two hands, you can either have them side-by side, on top of one another, or one above the other. In whichever scenario, have an idea in mind of where you're expecting the flow to go, otherwise the motion might be drawn between the polarities in your two hands. Your body responds to your intention/thought or your visualization of the action in this case of working with flows. If you hold with no intention or expectation, it may be less organized initially, but will then comply with its natural, inherent rhythm as the organizing principle applies its wisdom. Let your hands be soft and receptive.

If you're holding at the occiput, the expectation is to check the flow from there down through the spinal cord to the sacrum. In this case try to expand your awareness to include the entire spine as you hold at the occiput. Otherwise there might be a medial to lateral fluctuation, or the motion of the bones instead of fluids, which will vary depending upon where you are on the head. Higher up on the head in the posterior region, you will be in the area of the midbrain and posterior thalamus mentioned earlier which is a super highway of information passing to and from the brain, both sensory and motor.

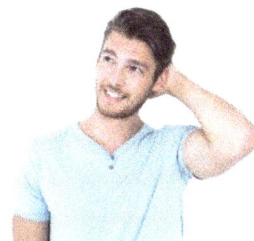

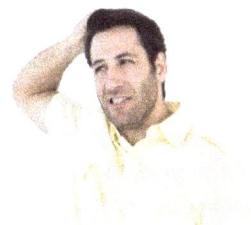

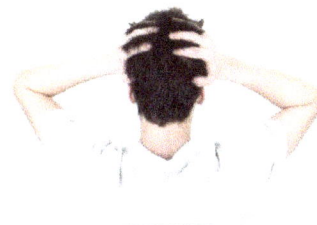

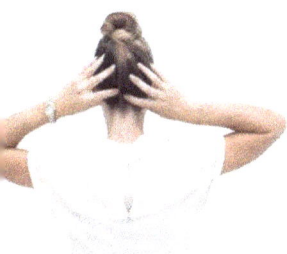

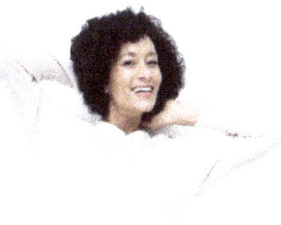

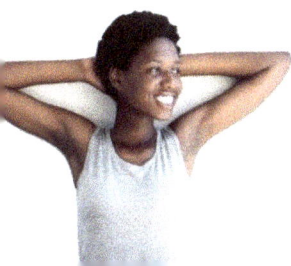

This region, near the most prominent bony structure (called the inion), is the location of Sutherland's fulcrum where he sensed the Breath of Life entering the brain and coursing through the cerebral spinal fluid. It is possible, particularly if your hands are on the larger side, to hold the base and inion at the same time, and you can experiment with the response of distinguishing them with your contact. Wherever you make contact at the head, and whenever feeling for the Tide, be super gentle and honoring, like you are holding an infant – something fragile and precious, because you are and it responds in kind.

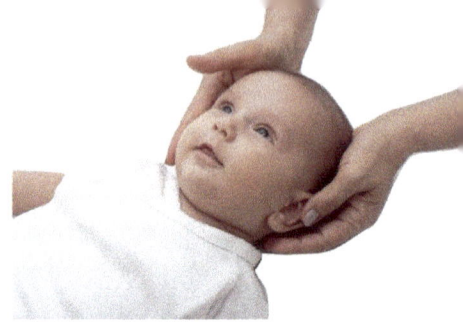

Also, the inion being the most prominent aspect of the skull in the rear, it will likely be the first to hit the surface that you fall onto and may be sensitive to the touch initially and for a while. If so, don't be shy to apply an ice pack there while those subcutaneous (greater occipital) nerves settle down. That being said, a very light touch here can have a wonderful effect on the release of endogenous endorphins – the body's natural painkillers – which can quickly shift the sensation of tenderness along with inhibiting the flow of fluids. You contact different systems depending upon the amount of pressure used, and there will be a different response in each case.

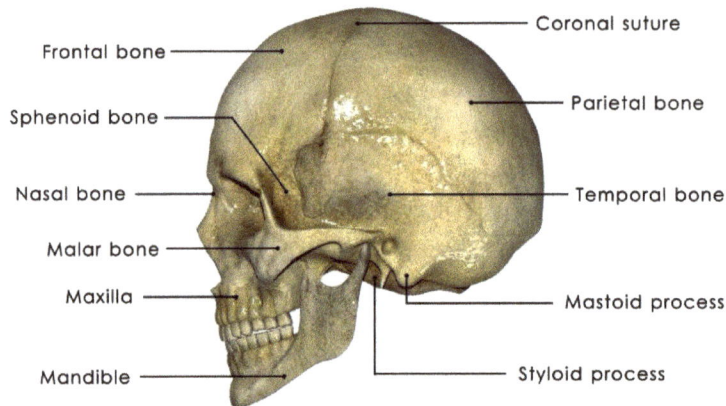

The occipital bone is just behind the mastoid under the parietal bone.

Remember the phenomenon of intra-osseous compression, whereby forces get stuck or held by bone within its matrix and it becomes contracted internally. With this gentle cradling and listening, you may feel the release of some of those internal forces followed by a widening of the bone as it opens and relaxes. There definitely is a situation where firm pressure/compression on the skull is called for and can call forth a wonderful shift in the membranes and consequently other systems underneath, but in this case to sense the fluids and settle the system, light pressure is best. The presence of your hands listening for fluid motion stimulates the flow of fluids that carry healing chemicals to treat inflammation, repair tissue, and clear debris. Stagnation is inimical to injury and to well-being in general, so opening the movement and flow wherever you can is fundamental, as Sutherland emphasized. Although the sutures are said to become fused early in life, Sutherland proved and many agree that there is a slight motion in all of the cranial bones, without which well-being is greatly compromised.

Sensing the eyes

The eyes often become sensitized after head trauma, and even after a long day at the computer, holding them for a few minutes can settle the sub-occipital area, the neck, face, hips, and feet, as well as the spine. Some like to palm their eyes, and I prefer to use my fingers; they're more sensitive to changes and pick up more information. Similar to the other areas palpated, the eyes will likely bounce around for a few seconds before they settle down, but be sure to use a very light touch so that they can move freely. See if there's a tendency for one eye to pull towards the nose or outward, and if it does, move one of your fingers to the nose or outer eye socket to neutralize those forces and release the eye back to its midline. One eye may be firmer than the other if you press lightly on it. If so, rest your fingertips on your eyebrows with the pinkies at the outer edges of the eye sockets if you feel comfortable doing so. Wait for a few seconds and check again. This won't apply to congenital displacements of the eye.

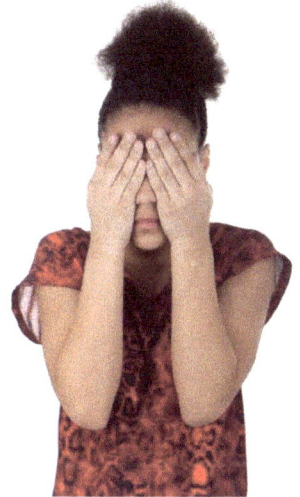

Sensing through the ears

The use of the ear canal in self-treating can be very beneficial as it serves to access those deeper regions of the throat where the buccopharyngeal fascia lives. It directly and indirectly influences many of the areas that become tightened in a fall, whiplash, or head trauma. This simple method can also give you an idea of whether or not your temporal bones are in sync. Although we are not perfectly symmetrical beings, it's still good to see in the case of membranous tissue around the delicate areas of the brain and throat that they can be as balanced as possible.

It's natural for some ear canals to be smaller than others, but you'll want to know if one side is smaller than the other due to an unnatural torsion due to tension fields that are creating the size or

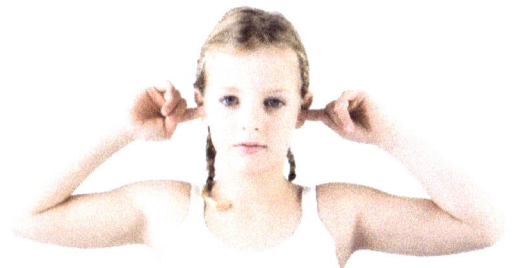

position difference. One way to see whether there is a rotation of the bone or fascia is to see if the hand positions are different when your fingers are in your ears. Check in the mirror and see if one palm is facing forward and the other slightly up or down. Sometimes you'll be able to feel the difference with your fingers. In this case, the little girl's palms are facing slightly different directions, and though we don't know exactly what she's doing with her fingers, the difference is marked enough that there probably is a change in the angle of the canal or the sync of the motion of the temporal bones.

Your fingers will be moving into the concha area of the outer ear, just inside the lobe structures and its inner cartilage into the 'foyer' so-to-speak of the ear canal – where you place the Q-tip when you want to clean your ears, but not pressing in farther than that. The posterior rim of this sector has a firmer wall than the anterior and so is easier to find a landmark upon. Once you hit that firm 'wall', back off a bit so you sense the interior fascia that connects it to the deeper regions of the throat. When you're there, at the right spot with the right pressure, if you move your fingers slightly you'll feel an echo in your throat. If the pressure is a little too much, the echo will be felt at the occiput. Hold there gently and let the organizing principle do the rest. It'll unwind places you'll never be able to touch with your hands, but the relief will spread and take pressures off deep, anterior and ventral portions of the brain stem.

Sensing the soft palate

Another way to access the fascia at the back of the throat is to manipulate the tongue, this time in a posterior direction. Earlier the exercise was to stick the tongue out, but this time the movement will be to retract the tongue as far back in your mouth as you can, applying some pressure to the hard palate while putting the soft palate and buccopharyngeal fascia into slack. The tongue is in a similar position as when you have a mouth full of food and it has to be displaced inferior and posterior. When you've reached the sweet spot with putting those tissues into ease, you'll feel the echo response all the way down the spine via the esophagus and possibly the dural tube. Releasing the deep, core areas not only support the healing process for whiplash and post-concussive residuals, but it ultimately also frees up energy through the core and helps you achieve more effortless, upright posture.

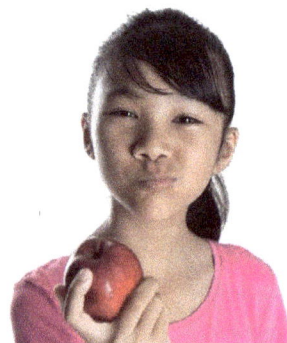

Explore, find the areas, the hand positions, and the combinations thereof that work best for your system. They work just as well for preventative maintenance as they do for corrective measures. The main thing is that you grow more and more familiar with your system and its tendencies, and with the Tide, its intelligent, organizing principle and your ability to stimulate and follow its movements. It is reported that the father of Osteopathy, A.T. Still said, *"All you do is begin a treatment, and the indwelling therapeutic forces finish it... This is not an ideology but a directly perceived reality that one begins to appreciate by following the therapeutic forces and accepting the wisdom behind the amount and direction of treatment. One must give up prioritizing by formulation and learn the deeper science of knowing the movements of life."* (An Osteopathic Odyssey, James Jealous, D.O., Tame Prepress, November 2015)

This indeed was my experience in each of these most recent explorations whereby the process led itself deeper and deeper into the inquiry, pointing to varying layers of the lesions, revealing what was holding them into the matrix, and bathing them with the Tidal fluids and energies that would both carry away the remnants of the injuries, and reset the tissue fields into their normal stasis. The Breath of Life continues opening, finding, releasing, and healing into itself, turning the process back into a spiritual one that removes restrictions to the deepening recognition of the Heart and inner Nature that creates, breathes, and animates all of its systems.

I'm both amazed and grateful for this process! I thank you for joining me in this exploration of the brain's mysterious mandala. I hope you feel inspired and encouraged to seek well-being in all the forms you feel resonance with. I also hope you'll share this message with those you feel could benefit from the information presented here. As for bowling, the blank spot in my brain has gone away not returned, there is no longer a pull up the arm into my neck and head that used to trigger symptoms, and my game continues to improve. I can't use post-concussive issues anymore as an excuse for my scores being all over the place, so consistency is still something to enjoy working toward. However, a gentleman came up to me the other day and said, "I don't want to jinx you, but you're the smoothest bowler I've ever seen; and I mean EVER!" I'll take that as a validation for the integration coming in more and more that opposes gravity.

www.ingramcontent.com/pod-product-compliance
Lightning Source LLC
Chambersburg PA
CBHW042350030426
42336CB00025B/3429